PRESCRIPTION DETOX

What people are saying about "Prescription Detox: How Our Allegiance to Big Pharma Makes Us Sicker and How You Can Heal Without Meds"

An absolute "must read" for those who want to take charge of their own health - naturally. With Cheryl Winter as your guide, your family, friends, and loved ones will be able to navigate major health challenges by searching for the underlying root cause without resorting to toxic drugs to suppress symptoms. Brilliant!!

Ann Louise Gittleman, Ph.D., C.N.S.
New York Times bestselling author of over 30 books on detox,
health and healing
Creator of Fat Flush

"Optimal health is true wealth! In order to enjoy both, one must understand what Cheryl clearly explains...that food is either medicine or poison! We can heal our bodies and keep them healthy by using food as medicine instead of prescription drugs."

Julie Beth Yelin, M.D.
Choose Health Wellness Center, PLLC

"Finally, someone is addressing the root problems of our "fat, sick, & nearly dead" society. I love how Cheryl goes straight to the causes of what is ailing us! Learning how to get rid of the foods that are making us sick is key to living a long and healthy life without prescription medications. This book is an easy read, and the steps she lays out are easy to follow. This is a must read for anyone wanting real solutions to re-gain their health.

Gail Clayton, R.Ph., M.S., CNS
Beyond Pharmaceuticals, LLC

As a wellness chef, I specialize in serving clients from practitioner to plate. Everyday, I receive phone calls from patients, who have been desperately failed by our healthcare system. In her new book titled *"Prescription Detox: How Our Allegiance to Big Pharma Makes Us Sicker and How You Can Heal Without Meds,"* Cheryl Winter boldly explains how conventional Western healthcare has failed its patients. Once a working member of this establishment, Cheryl could no longer participate in a sick-care system, writing prescriptions that only continued to harm her patients and never heal them. In a very authentic and conversational voice, Cheryl takes you on a journey to create health and wellness in your life. One that is not dependent on a pharmaceutical pill as its anchor, but rather one that involves true health emerging from the inside out."

Jacqueline Myers, Wellness Chef for Whole Food & Restorative Nutrition
GF Personal Chef | Gluten Free & Paleo Meals

"In my practice, I consult patients on hormones and using functional & integrative medicine to help them with disease prevention and illness transformation. The principles in this book are so valuable for my patients in multiple ways. Cheryl Winter has done a beautiful job in presenting her messages in such a way that all of us can use to better our health."

Van Tran, PharmD, RPh, FAARM, ABAAHP
Roberds Pharmacy, Conroe, TX

I have seen firsthand the impact that changing diet can have on a patient's health and wellbeing. If you want to transform your health and stay off of (or get off of) medications, you must follow the principles in this book! Cheryl Winter breaks it down in an easy-to-understand fashion. Her clinical knowledge and expertise are invaluable! My favorite thing that she says is, "food is the best medicine for the body." I am a believer. And I am excited to incorporate the principles outlined in this book into my practice!

Michelle Schneider, MSN, APRN, FNP-C
Owner-Optimal Hormone Health and Wellness, PLLC

Prescription Detox is truly a game-changer for your health. Cheryl tells her story first-hand on seeing the decline of patient health using solely medication, and how to finally get well with changing your diet and lifestyle. As a functional nutritionist, I regularly see patients in my office who have been told that they must take a medication for the rest of their life. Prescription Detox reminds us that we DO have control over our lives and our health outcome through the choices we make and the lifestyles we live.

Brooke Scheller, MS, CNS
Functional Nutritionist, BrookeScheller.com

As a Functional Medicine practitioner; it is exciting to see such an in-depth book on the topic of not just nutrition, but nutrition centered in a functional medicine approach. There is a significant difference! Cheryl's straightforwardness and timely approach regarding the chronic disease epidemic plaguing many people today is at a tipping point opportunity for those looking for a positive change in their health care needs. Most are fed up with being offered one pill after another, but never seeing any real results to move them into a state of wholeness. Cheryl's ability to convey this critical information within the covers of this book is simply going to provide you the tools you need to restore your health.

Debbie Hutchinson, CHHC, BS, MS
Functional Nutritionist & Founder of Turning Tides

"Finally, someone who has worked professionally for many years in the health care industry is telling the truth about the industry and the negative effect pharmaceutical medications can have on health! I have been in practice for over 10 years as a clinical nutritionist and have witnessed chronically ill patients taking 20+ medications regain their health and get off all their medications just by changing their diet. Cheryl is truly passionate about helping people live healthy and happy lives. The information that she provides in this book could very well change your life for the better!"

Danielle Heard, MS, MS, CNS, LDN, INHC
Artemis in the City, LLC

Cheryl Winter offers an insightful, practical and useful method for getting off medication and regaining your health. If you depend on meds to be healthy, this is a 'must read.'

Carlos Sanchez, PhD
Author, Speaker

Making complex topics understandable is the gift of a talented clinician. Cheryl's ABC concept embodies this. Starting with the basic idea of avoiding the toxins that make us sick and concluding with exactly what the body needs to heal. This ABC concept is guaranteed to give everyone from A-Z the results they desire.

Dr. Arland Hill, DC, MPH, DACBN
http://www.foodfunctionfreedom.com

If you're looking for a way to get off the prescription drug roller coaster this book is your answer. As both a registered dietitian/functional nutritionist and nurse practitioner, Cheryl is ideally qualified to help provide whole food strategies and solutions to wellness. I definitely plan to use this book in my own practice with my clients.

Mira Dessy, NE, BCHHP
The Ingredient Guru, Author The Pantry Principle: how to read the
label and understand what's really in your food

"After 20 years in the health care field, I have observed and experienced much of what Cheryl Winter describes in her book about the 'band aid' approach. This is a must read for patients who are sick of being sick and want real answers on how to reverse disease. The medical model that our health care system is based on treats disease, it does not reverse it. Healing starts with understanding how to help the body function optimally. Cheryl Winter not only gives a behind-the-scenes peek into the health care industry but also helpful tools to taking charge of your health and promoting wellness."

Tammy McGarvey, MSN, RN, FNP-BC
Board Certified Family Nurse Practitioner / Owner
Hope Family Health, NP PLLC

PRESCRIPTION DETOX

How Our Allegiance to Big Pharma Makes Us
Sicker and How You Can Heal Without Meds

CHERYL WINTER
MS APRN, FNP-BC, MS RDN, IFMCP

Edited by Donna Mosher
Published by JETLAUNCH.net

Disclaimer

The information presented in this book is based on the training and professional experience of the author. The recommended treatments in this book should not be taken without consulting your healthcare provider to be sure they are appropriate for you and your medical condition. Do not stop taking your pharmaceutical medications without first discussing it with your healthcare provider. Even when using relatively safe and natural treatments, appropriate laboratory and clinical monitoring is essential. This book was written for informational and educational purposes only and is not intended to treat, diagnose, or cure any condition. The goal of this book is to open your eyes so you can explore all potential options for health and wellness. The author and the publisher expressly disclaim all liability for any injury that may arise from the use of the information contained in this book.

To my one and only, my college sweetheart and husband of 37 years who has lovingly supported me throughout all my creative projects as well as educational and career endeavors.
You are my rock, Jerry Winter.

"He's the best physician that knows the worthlessness of the most medicines."

~ Benjamin Franklin

CONTENTS

APPENDICES

PREFACE

Health is Real Wealth

A person's wealth cannot be measured by the size or contents of their house, the designer of their wardrobe, or the number of dollars in their bank account. "Wealth is the ability to fully experience life," said Henry David Thoreau. Fully experiencing life can only occur when one is truly happy and healthy, and according to B.K.S. Iyengar, "in a state of complete harmony of the body, mind, and spirit, and when one is free from physical disabilities and mental distractions, the gates of the soul open." The loss of any part of this physical, mental, or spiritual health is a loss of happiness. Mahatma Gandhi said, "It is health which is real wealth and not pieces of gold and silver."

Too many are chasing material objects to enrich their lives, to the point that they have no disposable income to invest in real health care. Our conventional healthcare system is not real health care; it is disease-care. If you are lucky to have "so-called" healthcare insurance, you may refuse to pay out-of-pocket for items that will improve your health and enrich your life, assuming—incorrectly—that you are saving money. In fact, you are choosing not to optimize your health and thus your wealth, because health insurance is just that— "insurance." Health insurance pays for care when you are sick. Maintaining health and preventing illness–that's your personal responsibility. You wouldn't expect your auto insurance or homeowner's insurance to pay for your gasoline, household cleaning items, or routine maintenance; you purchase that insurance for catastrophic conditions. Only if we change how our society views health care will we follow the wisdom of Mahatma Gandhi and become truly healthy and wealthy.

ACKNOWLEDGEMENTS

I would like to recognize the many people who have helped make this book a reality:

Clint Arthur, my business and media coach who ended my procrastination and said, "Put a period at the end of your last sentence wherever you are, and publish this important manuscript now so no more people have to suffer."

Dr. Carlos Sanchez, my speaking coach, who provided inspiration, instilled self-confidence and provided me the tools to build a successful book.

Donna Mosher, my fabulous editor, who helped make my words clearer and more succinct, and for providing encouragement, support and dedication to this project beyond expectations.

Mira Dessy, my neighbor, friend, colleague, and author of "The Pantry Principle," who unselfishly shared her knowledge and book publishing experiences and resources.

To the many functional medicine leaders who have inspired me along the way, including Dr. Elizabeth Lipski, Dr. Peter Osborne, Dr. Mark Houston, Dr. Mark Hyman, Dr. Chris Kesser, Dr. Joseph Mercola, Dr. Isabella Wentz, Dr. Kara Fitzgerald, Dr. Aurora Romm, Dr. Arland Hill, Dr.Ron Grabowski, and so many more, and of course to all the amazing practitioners and teachers I have had the fortune to study under from the Institute for Functional Medicine.

Chris O'Byrne and his amazing team at JetLaunch, who brought this baby to life, from its vibrant and beautiful cover that portrays the message in this book perfectly, to the well-designed and artistic display of its contents.

To my family, my husband, Jerry and two daughters, Shannon and Heather, whom have supported me through the years, unconditionally, but who also sacrificed greatly while I studied to advance my career and pursue my thirst for health knowledge and desire to eliminate needless suffering in the world.

But most of all, I would like to acknowledge my patients who have suffered for so long needlessly, due to their trust in a healthcare and food delivery system that has let them down; suffer no more.

INTRODUCTION

The Prescription Med Epidemic

Before I became licensed to dispense pharmaceutical medications, I was a registered dietitian. I passionately believed in the power of nutrition and helping people improve their diets. I eagerly instructed them on a therapeutic diet that would help them restore their health. I spent hours individualizing a personalized meal plan for my patients. I loved what I was doing because I knew I was prescribing medicine (since I believe food is the best medicine for the body). I felt like an important member of my patients' healthcare team.

Unfortunately, this excitement faded after a few years when reality set in. It became obvious that doctors didn't see me as I did: as an important member of the healthcare team. To them I was on par with the lady in the hospital cafeteria. Most doctors were not ordering my services to help them improve their patients' health outcomes, but instead they called on me only to attend to their patients' hospital food complaints and poor meal service. And the patients didn't want to see a dietitian or be victims of what they considered dietary deprivation—they just wanted to take a pill.

This sad scenario is a reflection of what too many people experience in the U.S. healthcare system:

> *"I take Metformin for the diabetes caused by the Hydrochlorthiazide I take for high blood pressure, which I got from the Ambien I take for insomnia caused by the Xanax I take for the anxiety that I got from the Wellbutrin I take for chronic*

> *fatigue which I got from the Lipitor I take because I have*
> *a high cholesterol because a healthy diet and exercise with*
> *regular chiropractic care and superior nutritional supplements*
> *are just too much trouble!"*

Because our conventional healthcare system did not prioritize my services as a registered dietitian (because it wasn't reimbursable by insurance and therefore not profitable), and because doctors did not prioritize my services (because they never had a lick of nutrition courses in medical school to teach them the importance of food as medicine), I began to dread going to work every day. I knew I had to make a change. I deeply believed in the importance of what I was doing, but I felt defeated. I couldn't compete with the pharmaceutical industry. I couldn't change the system, so the system changed me, and I started a new career path that led me to become a legalized drug pusher. I was now part of the problem with healthcare.

The Centers for Disease Control (CDC) reports that chronic diseases (e.g. cardiovascular disease, diabetes, musculoskeletal diseases, depression, obesity, cancers), account for 70 percent of the disability and deaths of all Americans and for 75% of this country's annual healthcare costs. America ranks a mediocre 29th in the world for life expectancy, yet America leads the world in the development of new pharmaceutical drugs, as if they were the answer to health and wealth. Pharmaceutical drugs—I call them "legalized drugs"—may be making the pharmaceutical companies financially wealthy, but they certainly are not making the public healthy or wealthy. In fact, prescription drugs are the third leading cause of death in the U.S. and Europe after heart disease and cancer. But nearly 75 percent of physician-office visits result in the prescribing of pharmaceutical medications (legalized drugs), according to the CDC.

Do our doctors believe that pharmaceutical medications are the answer to health and wealth? Are our aliments and illnesses actually a deficiency of Metformin *or* Hydrochlorthiazide *or* Lipitor or (*insert name of drug*)? Seven out of ten Americans, according to a study published in the journal *Mayo Clinic Proceedings*, are taking at least one prescription medication. The most frequently physician-prescribed pharmaceutical medications are painkillers, cholesterol-lowering medications, medications to treat diabetes, and antidepressants. Shockingly, a growing number of people are taking all of these types of medications at the same time, and more!

I contend that the use of pharmaceutical medications is not the path to our health and wealth. Only the pharmaceutical industry is getting wealthy. It has been all too common for me to find my patients on ten or more prescription medications. If their diabetes condition is progressing and poorly controlled, they could be on three or four diabetes medications alone, plus painkillers if they were experiencing the complications of nerve pain after years of poorly managed diabetes. It is not uncommon for them to be on two or three blood pressure medications and two cholesterol medications, and most of my male patients are on a drug for erectile dysfunction. Despite (or because of) the use of these pharmaceutical medications that are supposed to make them healthy, the statistics prove that Americans are sicker than ever.

The first path to achieving optimum health and wealth (health is real wealth) is the realization that it is not a sprint, but a marathon. Achieving health and wealth is not a quick fix, as we Americans want to believe. But the pharmaceutical companies are all to happy to provide us quick fixes that are little more than band aids in the form of pharmaceutical medications. Sure, band aids are helpful in stopping immediate bleeding (e.g. the elevated blood sugar, elevated blood pressure, elevated cholesterol, depression, acid reflux, etc.). But if the band aids are used as the only treatment without addressing the real cause, then, all too often, the bleeding will worsen and more and more band aids become necessary.

Many times these band aids kindle the fire to create more and more destruction. What would happen if your automobile required oil, and you mistakenly put the oil in the gas tank? Obviously, the oil would be toxic to your gas line, despite the fact that your car needed oil. This is similar to what happens when we take pharmaceutical medications without addressing the real cause. Drugs of any kind are toxins. Simply covering up high blood sugar, for example, with a pharmaceutical diabetes medication does not change the fact that the body needs the right fuel to avoid the high blood sugar in the first place. If you keep taking a drug that is foreign to the body (like oil is foreign to your car's gas tank), your body eventually will combust. Your body may not combust today or tomorrow but over time it will malfunction to the point of no return, especially if it never received the proper fuel and maintenance it really needed.

As a family nurse practitioner working in the conventional healthcare system, over the years I began feeling like a legalized drug dealer, prescribing toxic substances under the mistaken belief that I was doing a good thing. I spent lots of money and time on my education, and time away from my family to be able to become a legalized drug dealer. You might compare those of us who prescribe pharmaceutical medications to a fireman. We extinguish fires all day and think we are saving lives and property. But why didn't I feel like I was saving lives? Don't get me wrong, I respect firemen and what they do very much, but once they have put out the fire, the poor homeowner is left to clean up the debris and destruction. In my case, the patient is left to deal with the side effects and adverse reactions from the pharmaceutical medication(s) and the continuance of the disease state because the real cause was never addressed.

Conventional healthcare has failed patients because we have made them believe that their health condition was due to a deficiency of a pharmaceutical medication. We in the healthcare industry are people pleasers. We want our patients to come back to us. After all, we need them to stay in business. All too often, we give them what they want: a pill. We know how hard it is to change lifestyle behaviors, and we don't want to inconvenience them. We don't have time to show patients what is needed to address the true cause(s) of their condition. We don't get paid to do that. And because we legalized drug dealers never told them what lifestyle behaviors could stop the on-going devastation, they falsely believed they were doing what their doctors wanted them to do by taking their medications every day at the right time without failure. We do have time to at least tell them that small amount of information, or we will delegate that task to our medical assistant so we can hurry up and prescribe more pharmaceutical drugs to the next patient.

Prescription drugs have become the inevitable expectations for Americans as they enter their golden years, however, even the young (our children, teens, and young adults) now expect a prescription medication for every ailment. Our society has become a population of prescription pill poppers. This is not an accident, I assure you. It is a well-calculated plan by the pharmaceutical industry. Its mission is not to rid the world of chronic illness, but to perpetuate it. For without illness, there is no money to be made in this very lucrative business. The pharmaceutical industry has higher profit margins than any other industry. Just turn on the television, and you will find one drug commercial after another. Those ads are not cheap.

Why so many commercials? Because there are so many drugs. Let's again take diabetes medications, for example. There are at least eleven classes of diabetes medications, and within each class there may be three to five different brands. Only different side effects distinguish them, thanks to the slight molecular manipulation made by the scientists so the medication can be patented as their own. Of course, each company is claiming their brand is better and that they found a better way to manage diabetes. Note, however, I said "manage" diabetes, not cure it. Wouldn't it be nice if a pharmaceutical company invested the billions of dollars they use to create a drug and bring it to market in finding a cure, rather than just to compete with an equivalent product already on the market? Of course it would be, but there is no money in finding a cure. Diabetes is one of the most profitable chronic conditions for the pharmaceutical industry, but I assure you, there are countless other diseases and conditions that are very profitable for pharmaceutical companies as well. Benevolence does not motivate pharmaceutical companies. They are motivated not for the good of consumers but to boost the company stock.

In fact, pharmaceutical companies are hurting this nation to its very core. As new prescription drugs are introduced and older drugs become available over the counter (OTC) or in generic formulations, self-medication has become commonplace, resulting in adverse reactions to drugs every day. Each year in the U.S., there are over 700,000 visits to hospital emergency departments because of adverse drug events from a single pharmaceutical medication or from combining pharmaceutical and over-the-counter medications. About one-third of adverse events during hospitalizations include a drug-related harm, leading to even longer hospital stays and greater expense. Each year, some two million cases of drug complications result in 180,000 deaths or life-threatening illnesses.

You might be asking, well, aren't the pharmaceutical companies under strict regulations from the FDA to assure good manufacturing and a quality drug while being transparent and providing the most honest and scientifically tested product? Well, the answer would be yes, absolutely, but in reality, they find a way to get around the loopholes. In 2013, GlaxoSmithKline agreed to pay the U.S. Department of Justice to settle $3 billion of civil and criminal charges related to misbranding of their drugs Paxil and Wellbutrin and their failure to disclose safety information about the diabetes medication Avadia. Even though this was the largest fine ever against a drug company, it was a drop in the bucket for them. It's common practice for pharmaceutical companies to set aside funds for such instances. It's cheaper to pay the fine than to lose the potential revenue—it's simply the cost of doing business. For any other type of company, these large sums would prove disastrous. But not for the pharmaceutical industry. They understand exactly what they are doing, so don't be fooled.

The manipulation by the pharmaceutical industry for mega profits starts even before the actual marketing of the drug. In some instances, it starts in the research lab. The bias in research studies conducted by pharmaceutical companies is well known in the medical scientific community. The drug companies are responsible for the research, not a third-party, unbiased scientist. Third-party research is rare and difficult to do without financial backing.

It's not unheard of for creative statisticians to fabricate an even more positive effect for a drug based on how they phrase certain risk benefits. For example, researchers and pharmaceutical companies often use "relative" risk statistics to report the results of drug studies. They might say, "in this trial, statins (cholesterol-lowering medications) reduced the risk of heart attack by 30 percent." But what they may not tell you is that the "absolute" (actual) risk of having a heart attack dropped from 0.5 percent to 0.35 percent. In other words, before you took the drug you had a 1 in 200 chance of having a heart attack; after taking the drug you have a 1 in 285 chance of having a heart attack. That's not nearly as impressive as using the 30 percent relative risk number, but it provides a more accurate picture of what the actual or "absolute" risk reduction is.

The rates of efficacy of a medication are determined by the NNT (numbers needed to treat). For a cholesterol medication, the NNT is approximately 100, which means for one person to receive the benefit of the medication, 100 people need to be taking the drug. That is an efficacy rate of 1 percent. When you take into account the side effects of taking a drug, is a 1 percent efficacy rate really worth it?

Don't doctors who are prescribing these drugs care? Why don't they just stop? Honestly, the doctors have lost control. Between the insurance companies telling them which drugs they can prescribe based on the best deal they were able to negotiate with the lowest bidding drug company to the pharmaceutical reps who are giving the doctors the only education they receive on how to treat a patient's condition with their drug, who is really in charge?

Your doctor may be too busy to read the (biased) journal articles on the most recent scientific study conducted by the drug company, but the drug rep is there to tell them all about it. Your doctor is too busy seeing a patient every ten minutes to think for him/herself anymore. Your doctor is too tired after a long day to engage in new scientific technology and advances. I can say this, because as a family nurse practitioner I have walked in their shoes, I have done everything a doctor has done, short of going to medical school. I have received in-depth education and training programs, and I am not afraid to say that I am far more qualified than most doctors to help you "prevent" illness (and never need band aids).

It wasn't until I quit my family nurse practitioner job and removed myself from this cattle-call medical environment that I was able to rededicate my career to patient health, immerse myself into the world of functional medicine, and figure out that we are addressing chronic disease all wrong in the conventional medical world. We do a great job with emergency and acute care illnesses in this country, but we fail dreadfully at resolving chronic disease. In fact, we are seeing more chronic diseases popping up than ever before, which is likely another reason we are seeing more and more pharmaceutical drugs being created.

We now find ourselves in a midst of a silent epidemic of autoimmune diseases. Autoimmune diseases occur when the body's immune system attacks itself—basically the immune system has gone awry. These include conditions like lupus, multiple sclerosis, type 1 diabetes, rheumatoid arthritis, fibromyalgia, and others. Autoimmune diseases have been around forever, but not to the degree we are seeing them now. In fact, we rarely hear about these diseases from the National Institutes of Health like we hear about heart disease, diabetes and cancer, but the number of cases is staggering. One in twelve Americans and one in nine women will develop an autoimmune disorder, and the numbers may be higher, because many are incorrectly diagnosed. By comparison, only one in twenty Americans will have heart disease and one in fourteen adults will have cancer at some time in their life. This means that you are more likely to get an autoimmune disease than you are of getting diabetes or cancer.

Why the rise in autoimmune disorders? There is overwhelming evidence that the rise in autoimmune conditions is the result of our exposure to more environmental toxins and chemicals than ever before. This will be further discussed in Chapter 1, but suffice to say, band aid prescription medications are not the answer and will only continue to make the autoimmune epidemic worse. Drugs don't address the root cause in autoimmune disorders any more than they do for the chronic health conditions we are more familiar with.

If this is all not bad enough, our overuse of prescription medications is causing "drug pollution," affecting everyone, not just those taking prescription medications. Our waterways in the United States contain residues of a multitude of drugs, including antidepressants, painkillers, diabetes medications, birth control pills, and other chemical compounds. The popular diabetes drug Metformin according to a report in the *Journal Sentinel of Milwaukee*, may be responsible for altering the hormonal systems of male fish in Lake Michigan, causing feminizing effects. Water pollution also contributes to chronic health problems, causing additional treatment with pharmaceutical drugs that end up in water treatment plants, rivers, and lakes. Thus a vicious cycle of toxic waste continues.

I entered the field of health care over thirty years ago to make people well (not keep them sick), but throughout my many years in the "conventional" healthcare system as a family nurse practitioner, I found that I was doing just the opposite. My patients were returning to me every three months for diabetes "management," but they were not getting better. I found myself adding one new medication after another to their already long list of prescription medications. They were having one serious complication or side effect after the other. I finally had enough of this "SICK" healthcare system. I could not consciously continue writing one diabetes, high blood pressure, or high cholesterol medication prescription after the other when I know there is a better way. I could not continue to be part of a system that makes people sicker and shortens their lives when I know there is a better prescription!

THE ABCS FOR HEALING WITHOUT MEDS

The better prescription is now in your hands: *PRESCRIPTION DETOX: How Our Allegiance to Big Pharma Makes Us Sicker and How You Can Heal Without Meds*. This prescription is as simple as understanding your ABCs, and it will be your path to long-term health and wealth. Simplifying this prescription into three fundamental principals will allow almost anyone to successfully reduce or completely avoid the use of pharmaceutical medications.

A is for "Assess/Avoidance/Ability"

You will learn "How Natural Detoxification Capacity is *Assessed*," "How to *Avoid* Toxic Exposure" and "How to Optimize Your Innate *Ability* to Detoxify and Eliminate Toxins." This has been the missing piece of the puzzle for far too long in our conventional healthcare system.

B is "Belly"

You will learn "How to Recognize the Culprits Causing *Belly* Fat" and therefore "How to Minimize *Belly* Fat." You will also learn "How to Feed Your *Belly*." Food is medicine, and medicine is food. You will be able to avoid or minimize pharmaceutical medications if you can conquer these principles.

C is "Cell"

You will learn "How to Find Clinical Imbalances in the *Cell*," "How Core Lab Testing Guides *Cell* Repair," and "How to Fix the *Cell* to Get Well." Your conventional healthcare provider doesn't know this valuable information. It's important "to test and not guess." Our cells are too fragile to throw just anything at them, such as toxic pharmaceutical medications. Understanding what they need first before treatment can occur is essential.

You will get more details about these ABCs throughout this book. I promise you that this book is going to over deliver. You will learn to avoid poisoning your cells and how to nourish them better so they can begin to repair. This will put you in a better position to wean from prescription medications (under your healthcare provider's guidance). Perhaps this book will help you avoid prescription medications altogether.

My wish is for you to regain your most valuable possession—your health—instead of being robbed of years of vitality and quality of life. How does that sound to you? If you follow the wisdom in this book, you will never again need to be concerned with how you are going to afford your medications and your health care when you enter your retirement years. You will never again suffer from the side effects and interactions of drugs that rob you of your energy and steal precious family time from you while you are laid up in bed in misery.

Don't waste another minute and another precious brain cell. Continue reading this book all the way through and get the facts now so you can protect your most valuable possession—your health. You also will protect the lives of your family members who won't have to watch you suffer, who won't have to be deprived of your absence in their lives, and whose economic future won't be threatened by a potential medical bankruptcy.

It's time, too, for all of America to be enlightened. This pharmaceutical medication farce cannot continue. Improper pharmaceutical medication use is ruining lives. Illnesses are not being truly addressed, while these medications cause more disrepair and lead to a vicious cycle requiring more medications. Families are being bankrupted, not just because of the expense of their medications, but because they don't get well and are too sick to work. Life has become dreaded, instead of a gift to be cherished. Don't let this happen to you and your family.

It is possible to discover the cause of an illness and reverse it without pharmaceutical medications. Functional medicine seeks the underlying causes of disease, using a systems-oriented approach and engaging both patient and practitioner in a therapeutic partnership. By shifting the traditional disease-centered focus of medical practice to a more patient-centered approach, functional medicine addresses the whole person, not just an isolated set of symptoms. Functional medicine practitioners spend time with their patients, listen to their histories, and look at the interactions among genetic, environmental, and lifestyle factors that can influence long-term health and complex, chronic disease. Functional medicine supports the unique expression of health and vitality for each individual. Does your doctor practice in this manner?

You may think that functional medicine is a new form of medicine, but it is one of the oldest forms of medicine known. Hippocrates of Kos (c.460-c.370 BC) was a Greek physician of the Age of Pericles (Classical Greece) and is considered one of the most outstanding figures in the history of medicine. He is referred to as the "Father of Modern Medicine" in recognition of his lasting contributions to the field as the founder of the Hippocratic School of Medicine. He is often quoted as saying:

> *"Your foods should be your 'remedies' and your 'remedies' shall be your foods."*

Historians, however, are still debating whether or not he actually made this and other related statements. Nonetheless, Hippocrates is credited with believing that diseases were caused naturally, not because of superstition and gods, but rather the product of environmental factors, diet, and living habits.

One of the first lessons we healthcare providers learn during our training is to "first, do no harm." Yet, every time we prescribe a pharmaceutical medication (a toxin) without addressing the cause of the problem, is the epitome of doing harm. Of course, pharmaceutical medications have their place and relevance. If I were in severe pain and natural pain relievers were ineffective, I would definitely want a pharmaceutical pain reliever. If I had a life-threatening infection, I would want an appropriate antibiotic. Pharmaceutical medications are appropriate for acute illnesses if there is no natural alternative. The problem, however, is when they are used chronically to treat symptoms without working to rid the body of the real cause.

Don't let the conventional medical system trap you into thinking pharmaceutical medications will bring you health. True health and happiness will never be found in a pharmaceutical drug container. I hope you will read this short book now to discover *PRESCRIPTION DETOX: How Our Allegiance to Big Pharma Makes Us Sicker and How You Can Heal Without Meds.*

Part 1: A is for Assess/ Avoidance/Ability

Not everyone responds to chemical exposure in the same way, and the health effects of many toxins have been significantly underestimated, despite clearance from industry and government. It should not be assumed that current industry and governmental safeguards protect human health from the adverse effects of ordinary chemical exposures in our everyday lives.

The "A" of the ABCs of *PRESCRIPTION DETOX: How Our Allegiance to Big Pharma Makes Us Sicker and How You Can Heal Without Meds,* involves understanding how to "**Assess** Your Natural Detoxification Capacity," how to "**Avoid** Toxic Exposure," and how to "Optimize Your Innate **Ability** to Detoxify and Eliminate Toxins."

In the Introduction, I discussed how environmental toxins and chemicals have been invading our lives, contributing to autoimmune conditions and complicating and increasing common chronic health conditions. Toxins are chemicals and metals present in our food and environment that can be absorbed by the body and cause harm to cells and organ systems. In other words, they are irritating substances that disrupt the functioning of the body. Toxins accelerate aging and can damage DNA. Toxins can create triggers (or turn substances in the body into triggers) that can create free radicals (harmful inflammatory forms of oxygen that get loose in the body). Toxicity increases the likelihood of developing a chronic health condition, including type 2 diabetes, obesity, hypothyroidism, depression, Parkinson's and other neurological concerns, cancer, high blood pressure, Alzheimer's disease, endocrine/hormonal issues (infertility), cardiovascular issues, and more. Overall malaise and poor energy are also common symptoms of those with toxicity.

Our exposure to synthetic environmental toxins is widespread, increasing, and is lifelong. According to the Environmental Working Group (EWG), an umbilical blood study of ten American-born babies showed the presence of 413 different chemical toxins. Of these chemicals, 154 chemicals were associated with hormone disruption, 186 chemicals were associated with infertility, 130 chemicals were involved with immune system disruption, and 158 were associated with neurotoxins.

It is believed that exposure to these toxins in utero (during fetal development) or during childhood may increase childhood leukemia and other childhood cancers, cause early female puberty, menstrual and ovarian irregularities, and attention-deficit hyperactivity disorder (ADHD). Pound for pound, children drink two and a half times more water, eat three to four times more food, and breathe twice as much air as adults. According to the National Health and Nutrition Examination Survey (NHANES) data, children with typical levels of pesticide exposure from eating pesticide-treated fruits and vegetables have a higher risk of developing ADHD. So, you can see our children, our future generations, are the most vulnerable.

Even in adults, small doses of these toxins, accumulated over decades, can have a cumulative effect and can increase the risk for prostate and breast cancer, early menopause, and neurological damage. It's no coincidence that illness and the perceived need for prescription medications correlate with the rise of our toxic exposures from chemicals, including:

* Herbicides
* Pesticides
* Antibiotics
* Hormones
* Artificial ingredients in foods

* Processed and refined foods
* Air pollution
* Water pollution
* Cosmetics and body care products
* Medications and drugs
* Caffeine and alcohol
* Vaccinations
* Household cleaning products
* Furnishings
* Cars
* Plastics and plasticizers
* Exhaust and cigarette smoke
* Electromagnetic fields
* Ionizing radiation

This list can go on and on.

In addition to the outside toxins we are exposed to, our bodies create toxic chemicals during the metabolism and breakdown of hormones, and the body even creates toxic chemicals as a result of stress. Even the bacteria (good and bad) that live within us have toxic by-products that need to be eliminated. The first steps in treating most any health condition are to reduce inflammation and eliminate toxins.

As you can imagine, complete avoidance of toxins is nearly impossible in our world today.

Toxins are ubiquitous. Exposure to and the bodily accumulation of many toxins is virtually unavoidable in the modern world.

However, despite this bleak outlook, assessing the body's natural detoxification capacity while understanding how the body works to remove toxins will provide us the ammunition we need to help the body do its job. Also, it is crucial that we know where these toxins are lurking so that we can avoid them as much as possible. And finally, knowing how to optimize the body to allow it to do the detoxification and elimination work that it was designed to do will go far in helping us minimize our cumulative toxin exposure over the years so that we can reduce our susceptibility to disease in today's very toxic society.

CHAPTER 1

Assess Your Natural Detoxification Capacity

"The sensitivity of the individual differentiates a poison from a remedy. The fundamental principle of toxicology is the individual's response to a dose."

-Stephen Gilbert, Ph.D.,
Director & Founder of the Institute of Neurotoxicology &
Neurological Disorders

Most bodies are able to detoxify until they no longer can. That may sound obvious, but at some point, all of us will succumb to being unable to detoxify efficiently. Some will succumb to it sooner than others. If there is an overload of toxins in the body for any reason—an undernourished body, a compromised digestive system, or over-exposure to a toxic substance—natural detoxification becomes less effective. The body does have its limits. If you think of your body as a bucket that is slowly, over the years, filling up with toxins, at some point, the bucket will overflow if there is no drain. Your body has a tipping point. One day you may be able to tolerate exposure to a hazardous chemical without issue, but the next day, your bucket overflows. You may experience subtle symptoms or severe reactions you have never experienced to such a degree.

Toxins are broken down in a process known as xenobiotic metabolism. Special enzyme pathways convert them from fat-soluble chemical compounds into water-soluble products that can then be eliminated by the body. As we age, liver volume and blood flow are decreased, so our capacity for metabolism is reduced by over 30 percent. Thus, in the elderly, toxins often reach higher levels and have prolonged half-lives (how long they hang around in the body).

The six organs involved in detoxification are the liver, gastrointestinal tract, kidneys, skin, lungs, and lymphatic system. The liver is the principle site of detoxification, which is a nutrient-dependent process. Therefore, anything that compromises the intake of the required nutrients (poor diet, poor nutrient absorption, poor digestion, poor elimination, toxins, or poor liver function, for example), will make detoxification more difficult. The liver acts as a filter, taking fat-soluble compounds (non-water soluble compounds) and transforming them into water-soluble compounds so they can be eliminated. If the liver is unable to handle toxins, the body will store the toxins in unhealthy tissue like the brain and the nervous system.

The liver has a lot of roles. It is an integral organ of digestion. It produces one quart of bile daily and metabolizes protein, fat, and carbohydrate from the diet. Seven and a half cups of blood pump through the liver every minute. The liver also filters viruses and bacteria from the blood and has a role in balancing blood sugar and in hormonal balance.

When the liver struggles, you might experience:

* a slowed digestion
* inability to digest fats
* slow or sluggish metabolism
* sugar cravings
* foggy brain
* migraines
* irritable bowel issues
* abdominal bloating
* fatigue
* aches and pains
* hormonal issues

* immune system issues
* thyroid issues

Metabolism of drugs, toxins, and other compounds occurs in the liver in two phases. Phase 1 reactions involve the formation of a new modified functional group (an intermediate metabolite), which is sometimes more toxic than the initial compound. If Phase 2 metabolic function is weak or unable to eliminate these toxic materials made by the body, they begin to build up and cause havoc. Phase 1, through several biochemical processes (oxidation, reduction, hydration, hydrolysis, dehalogenation), essentially takes the toxic compound and makes it sticky so that something can be added to it.

Phase 1 reactions require the following nutrients:

* B vitamins (riboflavin, niacin, pyridoxine, B12, folic acid, B12)
* glutathione (neutralizes free radicals, responsible for the synthesis of glutathione S-transferase enzyme)
* branch-chain amino acids (leucine, valine, isoleucine) antioxidants (e.g. milk thistle)
* flavonoids
* phospholipids
* carotenoids
* vitamin E
* vitamin C

In Phase 2, through even more biochemical processes (sulfation, glucuronidation, methylation, glutathione conjugation, acetylation, amino acid conjugation), enzymes convert the transformed "intermediate metabolites" into the water-soluble compounds for excretion via urine, bile, stool, sweat, and skin. Several nutrients are required during these processes:

* vitamin A
* vitamin C

* vitamin E
* selenium
* copper
* zinc
* manganese
* silymarin
* thiols
* CoQ10
* glutamine
* flavonoids
* glycine
* taurine
* cysteine

One dose of a toxin that is seemingly benign to one person can be toxic to another person. The dose makes the poison:

> *"The sensitivity of the individual differentiates a poison from a remedy. The fundamental principle of toxicology is the individual's response to a dose."*
> *–Stephen Gilbert (1997)*

As discussed above, a person's susceptibility to toxins is largely defined by their ability to biotransform (change the toxins into less harmful chemicals), detoxify, and eliminate both the toxins coming from the environment, as well as even the toxins that the body makes through metabolism. You may be aware of various detox diets and programs that people occasionally undertake to help them reboot; you even may have tried them.

But detoxing is something that we need to do every day to support our bodies, not just a few times a year. The impairment of health that leads to disease doesn't start the day the person gets symptoms. Instead, it is an on-going process over time. Small daily doses of multiple toxins can have a cumulative, detrimental effect on our biological pathways.

Disease Risk = Toxic Potency x Cumulative Exposure x Susceptibility

Also, these multiple toxins can be synergistic (producing a combined effect greater than the sum of their separate effects).

For example:
Cigarette smoking: 10 times risk of lung cancer
Asbestos exposure: 5 times risk of lung cancer
Smoking + asbestos: 55 times risk of lung cancer

Alex, a 58-year-old business analyst, divorced obese male, first presented with fatigue, tingling in his feet, high cholesterol, and reported being told by a doctor that he was approaching a borderline diabetic diagnosis and was told to lose weight. He was a smoker for twenty-five years but quit ten years earlier. A detailed functional assessment of Alex's lifestyle revealed that he drank one to two alcoholic drinks per day, played golf at least three times per week, and ate bar food almost daily. For several years during and after his college years, Alex worked in a hardware store. Lab testing did reveal elevated markers for insulin resistance and at least a three-month evidence of elevated blood sugar hovering in the diabetic range.

Let's take the case of Alex, above. If Alex went to a conventional medicine physician, Alex would likely be prescribed Metformin, a "standard of care" initial diabetes pharmaceutical medication to reduce his blood sugar levels. The doctor would tell him to stop drinking and improve his diet. I am afraid that Alex might simply hear "take this pill" and lose weight without getting the proper tools to lose weight. All too often, people fall into the trap of taking even more pharmaceutical medication for the purpose of quick weight loss. This only adds more fuel to the fire, and it doesn't address the cause. Alex's current health conditions will not be resolved simply by taking more pills.

> *Health care providers need to consider that exposure or bioaccumulation of toxins may play a role in their patient's presenting concerns.*

So, why don't most doctors understand this?

*   They are clueless to the link of toxins to disease.
*   They know only their specialty organ system and ignore how the body works as a whole system.
*   They don't know how to test for toxins.
*   They don't know how to remove accumulated toxins from the body.
*   They prescribe toxins (medications) for a living, so why would they stop?
*   It would take up too much of their time.
*   They can't bill insurance for it.
*   They never studied nutrition in school. They don't understand how food can be both a toxin source and a resource to remove them.

Regardless if your doctor of conventional medicine acknowledges that toxins are a problem, they are, and you need to become your own advocate for protecting your health. As a practitioner helping my clients reverse and eliminate chronic disease without the use of pharmaceutical medications, it is of utmost priority that I assess their natural detoxification capacity, optimize their ability to detoxify and eliminate toxins, and help them reduce their toxic load instead of reaching for a prescription pad. Here's how I would begin to assess Alex's natural detoxification capacity and his exposure to toxins.

Step One: Identify Toxic Sources

Identifying toxic sources can be done in several ways, including actual diagnostic testing via blood or urine. The most important heavy metals to screen for are arsenic, cadmium, lead, and mercury. Exposure to the pesticide glyphosate should also be investigated, along with many other sources (see Chapter 2). Lab testing, however, is not the only way. A detailed toxicity history will provide lots of clues to potential toxic exposure. For someone like Alex, however, even without testing, I can glean several clues from his story that suggest a multitude of toxins have been accumulating in his body for a very long time and could finally have accumulated to the point of toxicity. For example:

Clue 1: His age. Of course, the older one is, the more toxins will accumulate, but Alex grew up when leaded gasoline was common (before it was outlawed). Accompanying his parents to the gas pump would have exposed him to this toxin for several years. Also, Alex may still have a mouthful of mercury fillings, which are now known to be extremely toxic to health. Before any detoxification plan is ordered for Alex, safe removal of any dental amalgams by a biological dentist would be warranted.

Clue 2: His smoking history. Cigarette smoke contains over four thousand chemicals, more than forty known carcinogens, and four hundred other toxins, including ammonia, formaldehyde, arsenic, cadmium, and hydrogen cyanide, to name a few. Even though Alex is no longer a smoker (which is great news), he still has toxins in his body that have accumulated over the years as a result of this behavior.

Clue 3: His alcohol history. Chronic daily exposure to the byproducts of alcohol metabolism plus the detrimental effects of alcohol on the liver detoxification pathways, leave him susceptible to poor biotransformation of normal daily toxin exposure.

Clue 4: Years of working at a hardware store. It seems innocent enough, but there are significant toxic exposures at a hardware store, including formaldehyde in plywood, lead in paint, dioxin in varnishes, and glyphosate in weed killer, to name a few.

Clue 5: Avid golfer. Pesticides keep golf courses lush and beautiful. Atrazine and other chemicals used in golf course landscaping are known endocrine disruptors affecting hormone metabolism; insulin is a hormone. Since Alex plays golf at least three times a week, he may be playing when the course has been freshly sprayed, thereby compounding his exposure.

Clue 6: Bar food/divorced: Because Alex doesn't cook much for himself and is exposed to harmful food ingredients on a daily basis, he does not eat healthy foods that would improve his ability to biotransform the normal daily exposure to toxins.

Clue 7: High cholesterol. Contrary to belief, high cholesterol is not necessarily bad. Cholesterol protects the body from inflammation and toxicity, and if it is elevated, it means it is on the job working hard to help us get rid of the invader. If cholesterol becomes oxidized by too many virulent free radicals, it becomes dangerous. More testing is needed to determine if Alex's cholesterol is oxidized. Because other clues indicate that Alex is very toxic, his cholesterol likely is too.

Clue 8: Obesity. Toxins often accumulate in fat stores. This makes for some angry fat, leading to insulin resistance and poor blood sugar control. In addition, because he is obese, Alex's diet is likely insufficient in the nutrients the liver needs to detoxify effectively. If there is also a problem with his gastrointestinal system (which is likely, due to his poor diet), it will be unable to eliminate the toxins, and the toxins will then be reabsorbed.

Clue 9: Elevated blood sugar. Alex's high blood sugar may have many causes, and toxic exposure cannot be ruled out.

Step Two: <u>**Assess Nutritional Status**</u> <u>through Micronutrient</u> <u>Diagnostic Testing and a Nutritionally Focused Interview</u>

The detoxification process is energy-dependent, and the proper type and amount of nutrients fuel this process. Nutrient deficiencies are a silent epidemic in the U.S. The standard American diet (SAD) has created a different kind of malnutrition than you may see in third world countries. Americans may not be getting nutritional deficiency diseases of the past like scurvy, pellagra, or rickets, but data from the Centers for Disease Control and Prevention show how prevalent nutrient deficiencies are among Americans:

* 90 million are deficient in vitamin D
* 30 million are deficient in vitamin B6
* 18 million are deficient in vitamin B12
* 16 million are deficient in vitamin C
* 8 million women have very low iron levels (Latinos: 12 percent; black women: 16 percent)
* 7 to 10 percent of children ages one to five are iron-deficient
* Women aged twenty-five to thirty-nine have borderline iodine insufficiency

These nutrients play a huge role in the detoxification process, and if they are unavailable to the body, toxins will accumulate, and disease and disability will ensue.

Step Three: <u>**Assess the Gastrointestinal System**</u> <u>through Test-</u> <u>ing and Review of Symptoms</u>

Once the liver has completed the two phases of detoxification, gastrointestinal tract must "take out the trash." The intestinal mucosa (lining of the intestine) and intestinal bacteria continue the detoxification started by the liver, making a healthy microbiome (the unique collection of gut flora that inhabits our intestines, influences our immunity, mental health, detoxification, and hormones) and daily bowel movements critical to the detoxification process.

If there is a problem with the gastrointestinal system, the body cannot eliminate the toxins, and the toxins will then be reabsorbed, which is why it is so important to "start with the gut." The gut should be the first body system assessed for any health complaint.

Step Four: Assess Sleep Hygiene

Proper rest is an essential element of detoxification. Unfortunately, according to the National Sleep Foundation, 50 percent of all Americans are sleep deprived, 60 percent sleep less than seven hours per night, and 56 percent report daytime drowsiness. In addition to reducing the ability of the body to detoxify, sleep deprivation lowers metabolism and leads to cortisol production, which increases stress and causes hunger. A reduction in the production of growth hormone and, consequently, decreased muscle mass are also consequences of lack of sleep, as is forgetfulness and low serotonin levels (affecting mood and food cravings). With insufficient sleep, the body also senses it is under attack and stimulates a chronic inflammatory response, which is linked to heart disease, high blood pressure, diabetes, and arthritis, to name a few. What if you could reduce or eliminate a blood pressure medication, just by getting more sleep?

Step Five: Assess Stress Management Habits

For most people, stress is the largest contributor to toxic overload; management of stress is crucial for optimizing detoxification pathways. Stress impacts our physiology and psychology, ultimately changing our eating and lifestyle behaviors, and vice versa. Prolonged stress can lead to exhaustion of the adrenal glands, which play a critical role in helping deal with stress. Adrenal exhaustion becomes a vicious cycle that includes depression, fatigue, feelings of anxiety, and lowered resistance to illness. Healthy stress-management techniques prevent adrenal exhaustion, which ultimately facilitates detoxification.

Step Six: Assessing the Ability to Move

Physical activity improves the detoxification pathways. Sweating is an excellent way to rid the body of toxins. Movement also improves the physical, spiritual, and emotional aspects of the mind-body, generating a greater sense of well being, accompanied by increased energy, improved sleep, and superior coping skills.

> *"Movement is a medicine for creating change in a person's physical, emotional, and mental states."*
>
> ~ *Carol Welch*

> *"Energy moves in waves, waves move in patterns, patterns move in rhythms. A human being is just that: energy, waves, patterns, rhythms. Nothing more. Nothing less. A dance."*
>
> ~ *Gabrielle Roth*

Step Seven: Assessing the Mind-Body

The physical, spiritual, emotional, and social relationships make up the mind-body consciousness. A healthy mind-body often coincides with successful stress management, including calming the mind and the body through relaxation techniques like meditation, breathing, or prayer. Starting off with just five minutes a day of a particular consistent practice will go a long way to reducing stress. Peace and quiet are so uncommon these days! It is often necessary, when feeling stressed, to close yourself off from all outside distractions and noise for a while. This will help you focus your mind and reduce your stress levels. Similarly, the healing powers of music cannot be ignored. Find a genre that makes you feel good and heals you.

Step Eight: <u>Assessing Daily Detoxification Habits</u>

Most toxins are unavoidable, and therefore, specific supplements and specific foods should be ingested on a daily basis to prevent specific or broad-spectrum toxic build-up. (See Chapter 3).

Remember:

> *Total Toxic Load Results from Total Toxic Exposure Minus Ability to Biotransform & Excrete Toxins*

Therefore, to reduce our total toxic load, we want to avoid exposure and optimize our ability to detoxify and eliminate toxins from the body.

CHAPTER 2

Avoid Toxic Exposure

"We need to accept the seemingly obvious fact that a toxic environment can make people sick and that no amount of medical intervention can protect us."
~Dr. Andrew Weil, Pioneer of Integrative Medicine

A toxic storm has reached gale force for each and every one of us. Environmental toxins, chemicals that we are exposed to in small amounts every day, are creating havoc on all our body cells. These toxins influence every single health condition people struggle with: weight gain, obesity, thyroid disease, diabetes, cancers, fatigue, allergies, hormonal imbalance, infertility, autoimmunity, autism, attention-deficit hyperactivity disorder, and more. Yes: these toxins exacerbate every health problem.

The number of toxins we are exposed to every day is daunting, to say the least. It's not a question of IF you are toxic, but how much. It's beyond the scope of this book to discuss every known environmental toxin we are being exposed to, but I will briefly discuss ten most commonly found in our toxic-soup environment.

Lead: Unfortunately, lead toxicity is common. As we learned from the Flint water contamination crisis, lead can leach into the water running through older municipal water lines soldered with lead. Lead was once an ingredient in gasoline and paint, and it still is ubiquitous in the petrochemical and battery industries. As mentioned in the case of Alex in the previous chapter, people growing up in the 1950s and 60s are commonly referred to as the lead generation. Lead is stored in the bones after it displaces calcium and iron. Women are especially vulnerable as they begin to lose bone mass after age 35. If there is a significant exposure over the years, lead will eventually enter the bloodstream. Women can even pass the lead through the placenta to their unborn child.

Common sources: indoor dust, cosmetics (e.g. lipsticks), gasoline, water crystals, toys made in China, lead pipes, ceramics with low-fire lead glazes, rice from China, wild game shot with lead bullets, wine.

Symptoms of toxicity: anemia and fatigue because lead displaces the nutrients zinc, selenium, chromium, calcium, and iron; cardio-vascular inflammation and hypertension; learning disorders, brain damage, and kidney problems

Practices to aid clearance: vitamin D, exercise, eating greens

Mercury: Because it displaces sulfur compounds that are needed in the body for detoxification, mercury toxicity can make it difficult for the body to excrete toxins via the liver or kidneys. Mercury displaces other nutrients, including zinc, copper, magnesium, calcium, and iron, appearing through micronutrient testing as a deficiency in these nutrients.

Common sources: certain fish, especially king mackerel, marlin, orange roughy, shark, swordfish, tilefish, ahi tuna, bigeye tuna; coal-burning plants, amalgams, vaccines

Symptoms of toxicity: a metallic taste in the mouth, anxiety, depression, brain fog, fatigue, body odor (from sweating out mercury), hormone disruption leading to an abnormal menstrual cycle, ringing in the ears

Practices to aid clearance: alkalize the urine with a magnesium or potassium supplement to boost clearance; selenium supplementation

Arsenic: Arsenic poisoning is a very common problem. A natural element of the earth's crust, it is found organically in soil and water. Inorganic arsenic (manufactured) is found in fertilizers and pesticides

Common sources: water supply, groundwater, chicken, shellfish, rice and grain crops grown in contaminated water or soil

Symptoms of toxicity: high blood pressure, heart irregularities, muscle pain, nerve and brain damage, lung cancer; thiamine deficiency

Practices to aid clearance: turmeric, N-acetyl cysteine, chlorophyll, methylation support supplements (B vitamins to support critical functions in the body, such as thinking, repairing DNA, turning on and off genes, fighting infections, and getting rid of environmental toxins)

Cadmium: Cadmium is a toxic metal that occurs naturally in the environment. It is used in the electronics industry. In the body, cadmium can displace calcium, which leads to softening of the bones, and zinc. It also can cause thyroid and kidney diseases.

Common sources: rice, shellfish, organ meat, cigarette smoke, electronics, plastics, fertilizers, crops grown in soil or water, pesticide spray, air, costume jewelry, children's jewelry, drinking glasses with painted designs

Symptoms of toxicity: bone loss, fatigue, kidney and liver damage, joint pain, shortness of breath, brain fog, dizziness, headaches

Practices to aid clearance: alkalize the urine with a magnesium or potassium supplement to boost clearance; sweat

Bisphenol A (BPA): BPA is an industrial chemical used since the 1960s to make certain plastics and resins; it is the most common toxin in the environment. Research shows that it can seep into food or beverages from containers that are lined with BPA. (Avoid canned products or use those in cans that are BPA-free.) It is also considered to be a persistent organic pollutant (POP); POPs maintain their activity in the environment, without breaking down, for a very long time. POPs are linked to breast and other cancers, reproductive problems, obesity, early puberty, and heart disease. Thermal paper, which most receipts are printed on, is often coated with BPA, so best to say no to receipts and have them emailed to you, if possible.

Glyphosate: Glyphosate is the active ingredient found in Roundup and other commercial herbicides (weed killers). We are being exposed to high amounts through the consumption of genetically modified foods that are engineered to survive the toxicity when sprayed with this common weed killer. Research now shows that glyphosate kills beneficial bacteria in the environment, in the intestinal tracts of farm animals (that we eat), and in the human gut in the same way it kills weeds. Glyphosate leads to antioxidant and mineral deficiencies like zinc and selenium, needed for proper thyroid function.

Common sources: alfalfa, canola, corn, cotton, sorghum, soybeans, wheat, sugar beets, sugarcane, oats, maize, sunflowers, potatoes, legumes—virtually everything, including our meat, since the animals are consuming grains

Glufosinate: Glufosinate is another broad-spectrum herbicide used to control weeds; like glyphosate, it is used on genetically modified crops and often as a pre-harvest desiccant.

Common sources: rice, spinach, peas, corn, radish, canola, wheat, beans, carrots, potatoes, barley, cottonseed oil

Transglutaminase: Transglutaminase, which chefs call "meat glue," is an enzyme that degrades protein and is used to glue meat pieces together to mimic a larger cut of meat. Used in restaurants and the meat industry, transglutaminase can be a problem for people who react to gluten and exacerbate problems related to gut hyperpermeability (leaky gut). If bacteria contaminate the smaller pieces of meat and become trapped inside the larger piece of meat, cooking will not kill the bacteria. Meat glue is found in non-meat products also.

Common sources: pork, fish products, imitation crab, processed meat, lamb, chicken, egg yolks (in restaurants), mixing dough, and store-bought meat tenderizer. Transglutaminase may be used to make dairy thicker and creamier and added to increase the yield of tofu (already made from toxic GMO soybeans).

Symptoms of toxicity: bloating, gas, diarrhea.

Atrazine: Atrazine is one of the most widely used herbicides in the U.S. Sadly, it has been found in 94 percent of the drinking water tested by the USDA, more than any other pesticide. It is most commonly used for corn products with the intention of killing weeds. You do not have to eat corn to be exposed to atrazine, however, since so many products are made with corn, including baking powder, ethanol, maltodextrin, cornmeal, corn oil, cornstarch, corn syrup, dextrose and dextrin, modified food starch, MSG (monosodium glutamate), starch, hydrolyzed vegetable protein. In addition to corn and corn byproducts, atrazine is found in sorghum, lupine, wheat, green onions, lettuce, cucumber, catfish, canola, blueberries, watermelon, eucalyptus, and other fruits and vegetables. Atrazine speeds up the aging process and makes you appear older than you are. Like most toxins, atrazine increases inflammation, which also leads to acceleration of the aging process. Also, atrazine is a hormone disruptor, causing hormones to become imbalanced.

Aluminum: Aluminum, the most abundant metal in the earth's crust, is found in many consumer products: beverage cans, aluminum foil, pots and pans, canned goods, water bottles, and deodorant. It is found in foods (anti-caking agents, coloring agents, emulsifiers, baking powder, and sometimes soy-based infant formula), medications (antacids, buffered aspirin), cosmetics, and more. Evidence of low-dose exposure is downplayed, but research links long-term exposure to aluminum to bone diseases, respiratory ailments, nervous system and brain disorders, impaired iron absorption, Alzheimer's disease, and breast cancer.

Avoiding toxic exposure is critical to maintaining good health. To avoid these and other toxic exposures, you must:

1) Become informed and know where the toxins lurk.
2) "Take the trash out" regularly.

Where the Toxins Lurk

Food: Shift your food purchases and consumption to organic products as much as possible to reduce exposure to added hormones, pesticides, and fertilizers. Avoid genetically modified organisms (GMOs), non-organic foods, processed and refined foods, industrial seed oils, and high fructose corn syrup. (See Chapter 6 for how to feed the belly.)

It is most important to consume organic dairy products (milk, cheese, yogurt, ice cream, etc.) to avoid exposure to the genetically engineered recombinant growth hormone (rBGH or rBST). Refer to the Environmental Working Group (EWG) website to stay current about which fruits and vegetables are most important to eat organic (see Chapter 6). Free-range meats and eggs are desirable to purchase as organic.

Minimize the use of large fish (swordfish, tuna, etc.) as they are higher in mercury, and avoid conventional and farm-raised fish, which are heavily contaminated with PCBs and mercury. Wild Alaskan salmon is an ideal seafood to consume, as are sardines. For more information on mercury in fish, see the resource in Appendix 1.

Minimize eating out in restaurants where these principles are not practiced, which, unfortunately, is most everywhere. Processed and prepackaged foods are also a source of BPA and phthalates.

Dust: In a study of dust from twelve hundred U.S. homes, an average of more than five thousand species of bacteria and two thousand species of fungi were found in each home. Interesting was the fact that the microbial makeup of the dust varied according to the geography of the home, and its composition could be predicted based upon the gender of the household and if that household had cats or dogs. It wasn't necessarily the vast quantity of the bacteria and fungi found in the dust that was the health risk, however. The dust itself was mostly harmless; not harmless were the chemicals and other pollutants that collected in the dust.

There is also evidence that household dust can make one fat. Researchers found that certain materials in house dust activate a protein called PPAR-gamma (peroxisome proliferator-activated receptor gamma) involved in regulation of fat metabolism, cell proliferation, and cell death. Another study found that dust contained oleic acid, a substance in olive oil and vegetable oils that contributes to fat gain.

Other products in the home, including plastics, furniture, and electronics, contain potentially toxic chemicals that infiltrate the home's air and eventually settle into household dust. In addition to this "shedding" of chemicals, pollutants enter the home through open windows and on shoes. I hate to be a wet mop (pun intended), but it appears that good housekeeping skills (using safe cleaning supplies) are a prerequisite for living a healthy life. According to the EWG, *"Ordinary house dust is a complex mixture of generally yucky stuff—pet dander, fungal spores, tiny particles, soil tracked in on your feet, carpet fibers, human hair, and skin, you name it. It's also a place where harmful chemicals are found. One study by the Silent Spring Institute identified 66 endocrine-disrupting compounds in household dust tests, including flame retardants, home-use pesticides, and phthalates."*

Home Chemicals: Sadly, the U.S. government approves the use of an average of seven new industrial chemicals per day, with little or no safety testing, and does not regulate the safety of these products. Many of these industrial chemicals are foundational ingredients in our cosmetics and personal care products. According to the Environmental Working Group, there are more than ten thousand ingredients used in our cosmetics in the U.S. The Cosmetic Ingredient Review (CIR), an industry-appointed and -funded panel, has screened only 11 percent of these ingredients since it was established in 1976. The majority of ingredients in our cosmetic and personal care products have not been reviewed or tested for safety. The CIR contends that since each product contains such tiny amounts, they are not harmful. But we are not using just one product—we may use ten or more products a day. Multiplied over a lifetime, the use of toxic chemicals adds up and contributes to an overflowing bucket of exposure.

If this wasn't enough, the EWG reports that regulatory loopholes make it difficult for any consumer to read and understand labels on cosmetic products. The cosmetics industry is not required to use FDA's ingredient name convention guidelines; an ingredient in one product can be spelled and labeled differently in another product. Virtually any ingredient can be part of a "fragrance;" it doesn't have to be disclosed if the company claims it is a "trade secret." According to the EWG, phthalates, which are dangerous chemical toxins, were found in 75 percent of all products the group reviewed, but they were not listed on the label because they were hidden in the word "fragrance."

Choose non-toxic household cleaning, bath, beauty, and hygiene products. Avoid alcohol, sodium lauryl sulfate, parabens, phthalates, and other petrochemicals in hair products (including shampoo and colors). Search for a hair salon in your area that is environmentally minded; avoid using hair sprays, perfumes, or other hair care products that use synthetic fragrances. Use low-toxin makeup and skin creams. (Avoid products with phthalates, parabens, propylene glycol, alcohols, and fragrances.) Avoid dryer sheets and fabric softeners; they leave chemicals on your clothes that then rub into your skin. In general, skin care products from health food stores are a safer bet. Consider using antioxidant creams on your skin, low solvent products with CoQ10, and Vitamin C. Avoid antiperspirants and antacids with aluminum. Since virtually all antiperspirants contain aluminum, it may be advisable to minimize or discontinue use.

Avoid spraying pesticides or herbicides in your home or on your property. Use only green and low-VOC (volatile organic compounds) paints and products in a remodel or a new home. Avoid urea formaldehyde in building products. Avoid furniture with particle board, or buy used furniture that has had a chance to "off-gas." Let a new car off-gas by keeping the windows open. Minimize the amount of synthetic carpet in the home or use natural carpets and rugs. Take shoes off at the door to avoid bringing chemicals and pesticides into your home. Avoid mercury-containing thermometers and fluorescent light bulbs. Change the filter on your furnace every three months using the best allergy filter you can find. Dispose of older leaded glassware; remember that glassware from other countries still may contain lead. Be aware of older homes with leaded paint on the walls; have it professionally removed. (See Appendix 1 for clean home cleaning and cosmetic resources.)

Pollution: Be aware of air quality and avoid going outside when high levels of pollutants are present. (Seek out the weather reports.) Use caution in areas exposed to industries producing plastics and batteries using cadmium and other heavy metals. Because today's homes are so tightly sealed, indoor air may be more polluted than outside air; use high-quality HEPA filters with a charcoal filter to reduce inhaled pollens and toxins.

Dental Care: Avoid mercury amalgam fillings; to remove them safely, consult a qualified biological dentist. (Locate a local practitioner with the International Academy of Biological Dentistry and Medicine at iabdm.org.) Get second opinions on root canals. Avoid if possible having two different metals in adjacent teeth.

Smoking/Alcohol: Avoid all cigarette and cigar smoking and second-hand smoke; arsenic and cadmium are present in cigarettes. Minimize alcohol consumption. Seek assistance for alcohol or nicotine addiction.

Medications and Vaccines: Avoid unnecessary use. Use dietary and natural remedies before taking pharmaceutical products, including acetaminophen, ibuprofen, antibiotics, and hormonal treatments. Be aware that many vaccines, including the flu vaccine, may contain thimerosal, a mercury-containing compound used as a preservative. Ethylmercury, found in medical products, including influenza and tetanus vaccines, eardrops, and nasal sprays, is similarly toxic to humans.

Water: Regular consumption of unfiltered tap water can contribute significantly to the toxic load of your body, including arsenic, atrazine, lead, and chlorinated hydrocarbons. Water quality will vary from city to city, but in general, it is best to filter tap water with a multi-stage carbon filter or reverse osmosis filter. Be sure it is certified to remove atrazine. Filtering bath water may be even more important than for drinking since the skin is like a sponge and absorbs contaminants.

Avoid bottled water in soft plastic containers, as the chemicals in the plastic may leach into the water. Avoid drinking from plastic water bottles left in a hot car. Even BPA-free reusable plastic water containers may leach harmful chemicals. Do your research before you buy one. Mineral waters in glass bottles are generally safe unless there is a question of the quality of the source.

Drink approximately six to eight glasses of filtered water or healthy liquids each day. Use glass or ceramic as much as possible.

Plastics: Plastics can disrupt hormones in your body. Avoid plastic bottles and containers with the numbers 3, 6, or 7 on the bottom. Plastic "sippy cups" for the little ones should also be avoided. These plastics can leach chemicals into the food, juice, or water. Buy juices and water in glass containers when possible and store leftover food in glass. Minimize the use of cling wraps; try to use paper wraps. Avoid polyvinyl chloride (PVCs). Do not microwave in plastic containers. Minimize washing plastic containers in the dishwasher under high heat. Also, avoid the use of non-stick pots and pans. Trade in your plastic vinyl shower curtain with a fabric one. Reduce the purchases of plastic children toys, opting instead for products made of natural wood or fabric.

Electromagnetic Fields: Especially for people with headaches or regional pain, decrease exposure to low-level electromagnetic fields. Minimize cell phone use. Set your cell phone to airplane mode when sleeping. Minimize your use of portable phones at home and shift to corded phones. Move the clock radio away from the head of your bed. New cars are loaded with electronic devices; measure the EMFs before you buy one. Install a filter on your computer to minimize the screen's blue light emission at night. Hard-wire your internet access instead of using Wi-Fi. Do not use a laptop on your lap; purchase a stand to place between you and the laptop. Remove dimmer switches and fluorescent lights.

Take the Trash Out Regularly

Avoiding toxic exposure is the first of a two-step process. Next, you want to eliminate any toxins that infiltrate your body. Here are some ways to effectively detoxify your body.

The body produces its own toxins as it metabolizes food and other intakes. Optimal nutrition is the first step to promote health and support the body's efforts to remove harmful substances. Support that process with good bowel function and regular elimination, adequate digestion, and absorption of the proper nutrients, including fiber. We will discuss the value of periodic detox programs in Part 2.

Infrared saunas and regularly sweating can detoxify the body; perspiration is an excellent way to cleanse chemicals and metals from the body. Sauna therapy is not appropriate for everyone, however, since it can lead to a dangerous electrolyte imbalance in some; please consult your practitioner beforehand.

Manual therapies such as massage may be helpful in mobilizing and eliminating toxins from the body by stimulating the lymphatic system.

Exercise has been shown to enhance adipose tissue (fat cell) circulation and therefore increases the release of stored toxins. Cardiovascular exercise supports taking the trash out through sweating. Hot-room yoga is very beneficial, as is any and all forms of movement.

Drink enough fresh, clean water to help flush the kidneys and bladder through frequent urination.

Stress management is a surprising way to reduce the toxins in the body. The effects of stress create significant toxins confronting most people. Mind-body interventions can be effective in managing stress. Find ways to include them in daily routines.

Cleansing protocols are plentiful online, but not all are effective or safe. Seek consultation and guidance from a qualified clinician. Medical supervision is required for any detoxification protocol. Laxatives are not recommended. Before attempting any detoxification protocols, consider having your genes tested; this can be done through several different companies, e.g. 23andMe.com. The purpose is to identify any genetic mutations that might be present and contributing to impaired detoxification pathways.

CHAPTER 3

Optimize Your Innate Ability to Detoxify and Eliminate Toxins

"The best way to detoxify is to stop putting toxic things into the body and depend upon it's own mechanisms."
~Dr. Andrew Weil, pioneer of Integrative Medicine

When you properly nourish your body, adding in all that is good and removing the bad, you will optimize your ability to support your natural detoxification processes. Understanding the specific principles for "removing the bad" and "adding in the good" will support your ability to detoxify and eliminate toxins naturally.

The body undergoes two phases of detoxification. Key foods directly impact the mechanisms in each phase and thus improve the metabolic cleansing process and aid biotransformation. Specific foods and herbs aid the elimination of toxins and enhance the body's detoxification pathways. They even help mitigate damage to DNA by creating chemicals that scavenge the free radicals that proliferate as a result of toxins and detox problems. Free radicals damage cells, contribute to disease, and accelerating aging.

A food plan to optimize the two phases of detoxification and eliminate toxins incorporates natural and whole foods that support, modulate, induce, or inhibit various biological processes related to optimal detoxification and elimination.

PHASE I DETOXIFICATION

Remove the Bad: charbroiled meats, high caffeine- and alcohol-containing beverages

Minimize: grapefruit (naringenin), high saturated and hydrogenated fat diets, low animal protein or a lack of complete proteins

Add in the Good: cruciferous vegetables, diets adequate in protein (meat, fish, eggs) and plant-based foods that provide complementary essential amino acids

PHASE II DETOXIFICATION

Add in the Good:

* Alpha- and Beta-carotene rich foods (highest to lower): pumpkin, carrot, squash, spinach, sweet potato, collards, mustard greens, red peppers, chard, dandelion greens, cantaloupe, romaine lettuce
* Quercetin-rich foods: apple, onion, kale, cherry, red wine, extra virgin olive oil, beans, broccoli, tea
* High chrysin-and luteolin-rich foods: broccoli, chili pepper, celery, rosemary, honey
* High D-glucaric-acid rich foods: (highest to lowest): apple, grapefruit, alfalfa sprouts, broccoli, Brussels sprouts, adzuki beans, tomato, cauliflower, mung beans, cherries, apricots, spinach, oranges
* Citrus foods: grapefruit, orange, tangerine
* Watercress and turmeric (curcumin)
* Dietary plant fibers
* Magnesium-rich foods (highest to lowest): halibut, almond, cashew, soybean, spinach, oatmeal, potato, peanut, wheat bran, black-eyed peas, baked beans, brown rice, lentils, avocado, pinto beans
* Sulfur-rich foods (highest to lowest): scallop, lobster, crab, peanut, shrimp, veal, mussel, chicken, Brazil nuts, haddock,

sardine, cod, oyster, beef, dried peach, egg, turkey, almond, cheddar, Parmesan cheese, dried skim milk, spinach, onion, cabbage, Brussels sprouts, chickpeas, figs, beans/peas, leeks, endive, potato

* Folic acid-rich foods: liver, chicken giblets, egg yolk, dried beans, lentils, split peas, soybean, almonds, whole wheat, potato, sweet potato, spinach, beet root, Brussels sprouts, broccoli, cauliflower, kale, cabbage, bok choy, asparagus, banana, orange, peach
* B12-rich foods: liver, beef, chicken, pork, ham, fish, egg, milk, cheese, yogurt, clam, rainbow trout, salmon, haddock, tuna
* Cysteine-rich foods: duck, yogurt, egg yolk, whey protein, ricotta cheese, cottage cheese, yogurt, red pepper, garlic, onion, broccoli, Brussels sprouts, oat, granola, wheat germ, sprouted lentils

Additional Detox Boosters:

* Probiotics and fermented foods: help with detox by helping provide an appropriate microflora
* Flax seeds: contain lignans and help bind and eliminate toxic by-products through daily evacuation. Daily dose: 1 to 2 table-spoons, ground
* Leafy green vegetables: e.g. spinach, broccoli, Brussels sprouts, cabbage, kale, collards, contain glucosinolates, which break down into isothiocyanates; improves detoxification, while feeding the gut flora and allowing them to flourish. Also, the fiber content supports a good daily bowel movement. Daily dose: at least 2 cups
* Berries (organic): blueberries, red raspberries, strawberries, blackberries are health detox snacks high in antioxidants that protect the cells from damage. Daily dose: 1/2 to 2 cups
* Pomegranate: has three times the antioxidant effects of green tea and red wine; it improves detoxification of the liver and

helps balance cholesterol and blood sugar. Dose: 2 ounces of unsweetened juice concentrate mixed in 8 ounces of still or sparkling water

* Olive oil: taken in amounts of 2 to 4 tablespoons daily, will not increase your weight and will improve cholesterol levels and decrease nasty inflammatory chemicals made by the body called isoprostanes. Olive oil is rich in phenols that help give the body a power boost to produce chemicals like glutathione, the body's major antioxidant.

* Dark chocolate: in addition to improving mood and keeping blood pressure and cholesterol in check, is a great detoxifier. It's okay to eat a couple of ounces of dark chocolate daily, as long as it does not contain other ingredients like caramel, crèmes, etc., and is 72 percent cacao or higher.

* Turmeric: this bright yellow herb, used in Indian cooking for thousands of years, supports natural detox pathways. Curcumin is the most medicinally active part of the plant and is also a bile stimulant. A daily dose of 1000 to 2000 mg is encouraged.

* Dandelion: a bile stimulant and bile motility enhancer

* Green tea: in extract form, is a potent supplement for weight loss, hormonal balance, and detox. A typical daily dose is 200 mg of green tea catechins or 4 to 8 cups of green tea. If you are very sensitive to caffeine, this amount could cause insomnia and heart palpitations, so avoid it and try something else.

* Resveratrol: found in berries, grapes, and red wine. Helps with so many conditions from menstrual cramps to joint pain. Can also take a supplement of 10 to 25 mg daily.

* Artichoke leaf extract: a typical dose is 320 to 640 mg, three times a day.

* Milk thistle: an extract from flavonoids that acts as a great detoxifier; increases glutathione synthesis, prevents depletion of glutathione, protects the liver from damage, acts as

an antioxidant, increases the rate of liver tissue regeneration. It also has been shown to decrease fasting glucose levels in people with insulin-dependent diabetes associated with liver cirrhosis.

* <u>Antioxidants</u>: like vitamins C and E, zinc, selenium, and lipoic acid are needed for optimum detoxification processes.

<u>Spices</u>:

Before pharmaceutical medications were ever patented, our ancestors used plants for their ailments. It seems the healing power of these plants and their roots, leaves, flowers, stems, and seeds have been forgotten. Plants exert powerful actions on the body with fewer side effects than medications.

In addition to our "farmacy" of good wholesome food, our natural pharmacy should include the spice cabinet, and I am not talking about just salt and pepper. It's important to integrate spices of all kinds into the diet at every meal to avoid the use of prescription medications and improve detoxification. It's easy—just sprinkle marjoram into your potatoes, ginger in your rice, cinnamon in your tea, cayenne and allspice into salsa. Be adventurous.

Spices contain compounds that act on the same metabolic and biochemical pathways that pharmaceutical medications do but without the side effects. You can't see the powers of spices, but your body definitely feels them.

This is not a book about spices, or I would provide a great deal more information about them. Just know that you should incorporate them every day into every meal. Here are just a few spices known to fight disease and aid natural detoxification:

* <u>Allspice</u>: allergies, asthma, cough, diarrhea, flatulence, high blood pressure
* <u>Almonds</u>: high cholesterol, diabetes, cardiovascular disease, high blood pressure, obesity, stroke

* <u>Amchur</u>: benign prostatic hypertrophy, cancer, diabetes, periodontal disease, cardiovascular disease, thyroid
* <u>Aniseeds</u>: asthma, bad breath, colic, constipation, flatulence, ulcer, dehydration
* <u>Asafoetida</u>: cancer, flatulence, flu, irritable bowel syndrome (IBS)
* <u>Basil</u>: stress, cancer, cholesterol, conjunctivitis, diabetes, cardiovascular disease, malaria, pain
* <u>Bay leaves</u>: arthritis, cancer, diabetes, food poisoning, mosquito bites, ulcer, wounds
* <u>Black cumin</u>: immune decline, allergies, asthma, cancer, elevated low-density lipoproteins (LDL), dermatitis, eczema, epilepsy
* <u>Black pepper</u>: Alzheimer's disease, arthritis, cancer, constipation, depression, high blood pressure, memory loss, thyroid, hearing loss, vitiligo
* <u>Caraway</u>: cancer, elevated LDL, constipation, diabetes, food poisoning, heartburn, indigestion, tuberculosis
* <u>Cardamom</u>: asthma, bad breath, blood clots, colon cancer, diarrhea, cardiovascular disease, high blood pressure, indigestion, sinusitis, ulcer
* <u>Celery</u>: arthritis, elevated LDL, gout, high blood pressure, liver disease, menstrual cramps, stroke, ulcer, vaginal yeast infection
* <u>Chili</u>: arthritis, blood clots, cancer, elevated LDL, diabetes, headache, tension, cardiovascular disease, indigestion, overweight, neuropathy
* <u>Cinnamon</u>: cancer, elevated LDL, diabetes, food poisoning, cardiovascular disease, high blood pressure, stroke, ulcer, polycystic ovarian syndrome (PCOS)
* <u>Cloves</u>: bad breath, blood clots, cancer, cold sores, food poisoning, genital herpes, gingivitis, hepatitis C, ulcer, toothache
* <u>Cocoa</u>: Alzheimer's disease, elevated LDL, dementia, fatigue, cardiovascular disease, high blood pressure, memory loss, stroke

* <u>Coconuts</u>: acne, Alzheimer's disease, cancer, Crohn's disease, infection, overweight, pain, vaginal yeast infection
* <u>Coriander</u>: bloating, cardiovascular disease, colon cancer, diabetes, diarrhea, eczema, high blood pressure, inflammatory bowel disease, liver disease, psoriasis
* <u>Cumin</u>: cancer, diabetes, epilepsy, food poisoning, osteoporosis, tuberculosis
* <u>Curry leaf</u>: Alzheimer's disease, elevated LDL, colon cancer, diabetes, memory loss
* <u>Fennel</u>: Alzheimer's disease, arthritis, cancer, colitis, dementia, glaucoma, heart disease, high blood pressure, stroke
* <u>Fenugreek</u>: cancer, cataracts, elevated LDL, diabetes, gallstones, infection, insulin resistance (pre-diabetes), kidney stones, liver disease
* <u>Galangal</u>: allergies, arthritis, cancer, diabetes, ulcer
* <u>Garlic</u>: alopecia, benign prostatic hypertrophy, cancer, elevated LDL, colds, flu, diabetes, cardiovascular disease, sickle cell disease, stroke, wrinkles and aging
* <u>Ginger</u>: arthritis, asthma, cancer, elevated LDL, heart attack, heartburn, indigestion, nausea, stroke
* <u>Horseradish</u>: bronchitis, cancer, elevated LDL, ear infection, flu, pneumonia, sinusitis, urinary tract infection (UTI)
* <u>Juniper berry</u>: arthritis, osteoarthritis, rheumatoid arthritis, bronchitis, breast cancer, diabetes, fungal infection, heart failure, hemorrhoids, high blood pressure, kidney disease
* <u>Kokum</u>: cancer, indigestion, overweight, rash, ulcer
* <u>Lemongrass</u>: anxiety, cancer, elevated LDL, diabetes, epilepsy, insomnia, thrush, vaginal yeast infections
* <u>Marjoram</u>: Alzheimer's disease, blood clots, cancer, fungal infection, heart disease, indigestion, stroke, ulcer
* <u>Mint</u>: allergies, anxiety, breastfeeding problem, cancer, Chronic Obstructive Pulmonary Disease (COPD), menopause problems, nausea, stress, tooth decay, PCOS

* <u>Mustard seed</u>: benign prostatic hypertrophy, cancer, elevated LDL, COPD, diabetes, heart disease, insulin resistance
* <u>Nutmeg</u>: anxiety, cancer, elevated LDL, depression, diarrhea, epilepsy, memory loss, low libido
* <u>Onion</u>: allergies, benign prostatic hypertrophy, cancer, elevated LDL, diabetes, heart attack, heart disease, high blood pressure, osteoporosis, scars
* <u>Oregano</u>: age spots, Alzheimer's disease, cancer, elevated LDL, colitis, heart disease, parasitic infection, insulin resistance, liver disease, sore throat, thrush, yeast infections
* <u>Parsley</u>: cancer, diabetes, heart disease, ulcer
* <u>Pomegranate</u>: Alzheimer's disease, angina, arthritis, osteoarthritis, rheumatoid arthritis, atherosclerosis, cancer, colitis, diabetes, high blood pressure
* <u>Pumpkin seed</u>: anemia, arthritis, osteoarthritis, rheumatoid arthritis, benign prostatic hypertrophy, elevated LDL, heart disease, urinary incontinence
* <u>Rosemary</u>: anxiety, arthritis, osteoarthritis, rheumatoid arthritis, dermatitis, cancer, gout, depression, diabetes, heart disease, liver disease, memory loss, stress, ulcer
* <u>Saffron</u>: Alzheimer's disease, anxiety, insomnia, atherosclerosis, cancer, depression, infertility, memory loss, Parkinson's disease, premenstrual syndrome, macular degeneration
* <u>Sage</u>: Alzheimer's disease, anxiety, cancer, dermatitis, diabetes, eczema, heart disease, memory loss, psoriasis, sore throat
* <u>Sesame seed</u>: Alzheimer's disease, cancer, elevated LDL, heart disease, high blood pressure, Huntington's disease, wounds
* <u>Star anise</u>: cancer, cold sores, flu, Hepatitis B, HIV/AIDS, mononucleosis, septic shock, tooth decay
* <u>Tomato</u>: cancer, elevated LDL, dementia, heart disease, high blood pressure, infertility (male), osteoporosis, Parkinson's disease
* <u>Tamarind</u>: cancer, cataracts, elevated LDL, conjunctivitis, diabetes, eye infection, heart disease, high blood pressure

* <u>Thyme</u>: aging, alcohol abuse, cancer, bronchitis (acute), colitis, cough, flu, heart attack, bacterial infection, stroke, tooth decay
* <u>Turmeric</u>: acne, allergies, Alzheimer's disease, arthritis, osteoarthritis and rheumatoid arthritis, asthma, cancer, dermatitis, diabetes, depression, flatulence, itching, macular degeneration, Parkinson's, reflux, sore throat, yeast infections
* <u>Vanilla</u>: cancer, sickle cell disease
* <u>Wasabi</u>: blood clots, cancer, elevated LDL, eczema, food poisoning, osteoporosis, tooth decay, ulcer

Part 2: B is for Belly

"The food you eat can be either the safest and most powerful form of medicine or the slowest form of poison."
~ Dr. Ann Wigmore, Holistic Health Practitioner

The "B" of the ABCs of *PRESCRIPTION DETOX: How Our Allegiance to Big Pharma Makes Us Sicker and How You Can Heal Without Meds,* gives the belly (and the body) exactly what it needs and not what it doesn't need. The bonus is that you will minimize your belly fat. This is not a new concept. Hippocrates said it best: "Let food be thy medicine and medicine be thy food."

Every cell in the body requires nutrients to function properly. Food delivers information. It has a profound impact on physiology, conveying messages within the digestive system, metabolic processes, and cell signaling. Certain foods can help reduce inflammation, lower blood sugar and insulin levels, support detoxification pathways, improve cellular energy production, and improve body composition. Conversely, poor food choices can increase inflammation, raise blood sugar and insulin, increase body fat storage, fail to prevent muscle loss, and adversely affect cellular energy, detoxification, elimination, and hormone balance.

Give the body the wrong information, and it will eventually fail you. People's bodies are failing them every day. But modern medicine only treats symptoms, as if millions of Americans are suffering from deficiencies of *"insert medication name."* This couldn't be further from the truth.

According to the World Health Organization, worldwide obesity has more than doubled since 1980. In 2014, more than 1.9 billion adults were overweight, and of these, 600 million were obese. Most of the world's population live in countries where overweight and obesity kills more people than underweight.

*   In 1900, the average male weighed 133 pounds, the average female 122 pounds
*   In 2000, the average male weighed 166 pounds, the average female 144 pounds
*   In 1985, in eight states 10 percent of the population was obese.
*   In 2000, no states could claim such numbers.

Obesity causes more than 15 percent of preventable deaths in the United States, more than alcohol, toxins, motor vehicle accidents, gun-related deaths, drug abuse, and sexually transmitted diseases combined. In fact, 75 percent of all healthcare dollars goes to the maintenance or treatment of chronic metabolic disease, says pediatric endocrinologist Robert Lustig. If that sounds outrageous, consider that metabolic disease includes obesity, metabolic syndrome, diabetes, and their consequences, including heart disease and stroke.

Health Problems Resulting from an Increase in Obesity

*   Diabetes: type 2 and gestational diabetes; there is also an increase of type 2 in our children, a disease once only prevalent in adults
*   Cardiovascular diseases: hypertension, heart attack, stroke, hyperlipidemia, hypercholesterolemia, metabolic syndrome, coronary artery disease, congestive heart failure
*   Musculoskeletal diseases: osteoarthritis, gout, hyperuricemia, degenerative joint diseases, back pain
*   Cancer: breast, colon, prostate, endometrial
*   Restrictive pulmonary diseases: sleep apnea, chronic obstructive pulmonary disease

* <u>Mental</u>: eating disorders, depression, low self-esteem, psychological conditions,
* <u>Alzheimer's</u> disease, and dementia
* <u>Other</u>: premenstrual syndrome (PMS), infertility, menstrual irregularity, gallbladder disease (gallstones), insulin resistance, general fatigue, stress incontinence, heartburn, indigestion, gastric reflux, complications of pregnancy, hirsutism (excess body and facial hair), colds and flu due to poorly balanced diets, increased surgical risk, and more

Type 2 diabetes is a well-known obesity-related health condition: a preventable condition that can be reversed or prevented. The United States ranks third in the world for the prevalence of diabetes, with India and China slightly ahead. It is predicted that by the year 2050 one or even two out of three Americans will have diabetes. A person who is overweight has a 40 percent chance of developing diabetes, and sadly, half of people with diabetes have no idea they have it. Even people with insulin resistance (pre-diabetes), who have not yet converted to diabetes, have been found to have signs of retinopathy (a leading cause of blindness) and other major complications.

Weight loss? No one seems able to agree on the best way to lose weight. There are countless books and diets on the subject (including this book), yet we are a nation with an epidemic of obesity that has no relief in sight. In most cases, weight loss can fully reverse type 2 diabetes, as it can for many of the other health conditions listed above. Insulin resistance driving it springs from the abdominal adiposity, that is, the belly fat. Reducing belly fat reduces toxicity and the need for pharmaceutical medications. Yes, it is as simple as that.

You see, not all fat is equal. We store fat under our skin, called subcutaneous fat, and in the abdominal cavity, called abdominal or visceral fat. Visceral fat may be called a "spare tire" or a "beer gut" or "belly fat." The best way to distinguish subcutaneous fat from visceral fat is with a tape measure (not a scale). Your waist circumference is far more important than your body mass index (BMI) in predicting your risk for disease.

PRESCRIPTION DETOX: How Our Allegiance to Big Pharma Makes Us Sicker and How You Can Heal Without Meds, prescribes giving your belly (your body) more food, not more medicine. That's right! You thought I would say less food, didn't you? But Americans are not feeding their body "real" food. The food is often fake and full of foreign chemicals that the body cannot recognize. Your belly knows the difference between real, wholesome food and fake, processed foods. Your belly knows the difference between industrial fats and oils and natural oils and fats. Your belly doesn't know what to do with the excess sugar added to the fake foods intentionally formulated to addict us eating more. Your belly goes haywire, and it bulges with fat in places where fat doesn't belong.

Although we are a nation of food abundance and overweight, the belly (and therefore the body) is malnourished, despite the calorie overage it is receiving. Our soils have been depleted of the nutrients needed to grow nutritious crops. We spray those crops with pesticides that cause the disruption of human cell membranes and cell functioning. Nutrient deficiencies and environmental toxins compromise the ability of the immune system to combat foreign invaders and can lead to conditions of inflammation and even autoimmunity. We know, for example, that type 2 diabetes is a disease of inflammation. Considering the foreign toxins and food additives in the food supply that the body must contend with, type 2 diabetes also may be considered a condition caused by autoimmunity (the body attacking itself), like in other autoimmune conditions, including type 1 diabetes, rheumatoid arthritis, multiple sclerosis, lupus, ankylosing spondylitis, and more.

Most of our meat sources are institutionally farmed, fed genetically-modified (GMO) corn (contributing to our elevated blood sugars and insulin resistance), and pumped with hormones to make the animals grow faster and increase profits. Also, institutionally farmed animals are regularly injected with antibiotics to reduce the infections they get from being tightly confined and the illnesses that result from their unnatural diets. Fifty percent of all antibiotics go to big farm agriculture, so you know there is an absolute direct connection between the food and pharmaceutical medication industries. Antibiotic resistance today is rampant in our society; children are going through puberty sooner—something that was not seen when livestock was exclusively pasture-raised, getting their nourishment from naturally green leafy forage and not routinely given hormones or antibiotics.

Our processed restaurant and fast foods are full of sugar, additives, and artificial ingredients that are deficient in micronutrients, harmful to our human cells, and that promote insulin resistance, inflammation, and autoimmunity. When we add to this toxic-soup mix our significantly stressed lives, environmental toxins, poor diets, lack of sleep, overweight and inactivity... well, *bon appétit*! We have cooked up an inflammatory stew, wreaking havoc within every cell of the body, leading to inflammatory and autoimmune conditions that have caused the pharmaceutical industry to flood the market with more and more pharmaceutical medications, making you think that your illness is due to a deficiency of those meds.

Obviously, this lifestyle is not serving us well, and it's time to get back to the basics: eating real food grown without pesticides in nutrient-rich soil—not food from manmade packages and drive-through restaurants. We need to reduce—or eliminate—sugar and refined carbohydrates from our diets. We can reclaim the taste buds that were hijacked by the food manufacturing companies, which strategically sabotaged us to desire their deadly foods. It seems that the food manufacturing and pharmaceutical companies are in cahoots with each other to sabotage our lives for their financial gain. Ideally, it's time for us let go of our fast-paced lives, recapture our family time, play outside with our kids, and then show them where the kitchen is, and teach them how to cook real foods.

"People are fed by the food industry, which pays no attention to health, and are treated by the health industry, which pays no attention to food."
~ Wendell Berry

It may take a community to significantly change our food supply, but we can each make concerted efforts to properly nourish our children and our belly (body) by setting good examples for them. Most people say they know how to eat well—and they think they *are* eating well—yet we are a country of severely malnourished people. We have learner's manuals for our cars, our phones, and our computers. But we don't come with a manual on how to feed the belly (body), our most precious gift. In fact, people are confused about the different nutrition messages and whom to believe. Nutrition has become like religion and politics—everyone has an opinion, and you better not state your opinion unless you want a debate.

Nutrition is a concert, not a solo.
~ author unknown

Proper nutrition is not subject to opinion, and there should be no debate. Nutrition is biochemistry, and that is not an opinion, that is a fact. The body wants what the body wants. The body tells us how to take care of it and what it needs. It's time we paid attention to the biochemistry of the body and give it what it needs. If we load it with garbage in the form of poor food, stress, and sedentary lives, it will turn into a garbage dump. Garbage in: garbage out. It's time we make a concerted effort to help reduce the garbage and replenish our body and environment with wholesomeness and purity.

CHAPTER 4

Recognize the Culprits
Causing Belly Fat

*Every forkful we put into our mouth has the potential to be
either inflammatory or anti-inflammatory.*

Americans are facing an epidemic of obesity. The Centers for Disease Control and Prevention (CDC) report that nearly 40 percent of adults and 17 percent of teenagers are obese.

The cause of obesity and the accompanying excess belly fat is a complicated topic. Everyone claims they know what causes it and what to do about it, but if that is true, would this epidemic be so rampant? Fixing the epidemic of obesity is indeed the difficult part, but recognizing the cause is real obvious. The simple answer to the cause of excess belly fat is our "modern" lifestyle. This modern lifestyle includes an increased consumption of processed and refined foods, too much fructose (especially high-fructose corn syrup found in sodas, candy, and processed foods), too many grains (especially white flour), and too much industrial seed oils. (These are oils, including soy and canola that may be labeled "vegetable" oil.) And, of course, remember those environmental toxins, previously discussed.

And it is possible that the traditional medical community finally is catching on to the cause of this epidemic. The editors of the Journal of the American Medical Association (JAMA) have hinted that food might just be the source of obesity!

"The obesity epidemic in the United States is now three decades old, and huge investments have been made in research, clinical care, and development of various programs to counteract obesity," commented editors of JAMA. "However, few data suggest the epidemic is diminishing," they added.

"Perhaps it is time for an entirely different approach, one that emphasizes collaboration with the food and restaurant industries that are in part responsible for putting food on dinner tables." What a novel idea!

So yes, even conventional medicine is beginning to suspect that the food we eat as a result of our so-called modern lifestyle may be influencing obesity and belly fat.

Our modern lifestyle behaviors also contribute to obesity and belly fat. Consider the significant added stress most everyone seems to be dealing with, increasing sedentary behaviors and a lack of regular exercise, reduced quality sleep, infections, and dysregulated gut flora, which result from these impacts.

No one is completely immune to the negative impacts of our modern lifestyle, and the consequences result in three effects to the body:

1) Inflammation
2) Obesity
3) Activation of a genetic predisposition

Let's dissect each one of these more closely:

1) **Inflammation**:

You likely are familiar with the term "inflammation." You know that if you cut yourself or sprain an ankle, the area very quickly swells and becomes red and painful. That's "acute" inflammation: the body's effort to heal as quickly and efficiently as possible. This is a good and helpful thing. The term inflammation, from the Latin *inflammare* (to set on fire), was first used two thousand years ago by the Roman medical writer, Aulus Cornelius Celsus, who documented the four cardinal signs of inflammation: *rubor et tumor cum colore et dolore* (redness and swelling with heat and pain).

Two centuries later, the Greek physician Galen promoted the idea that inflammation, especially pus, was a beneficial response to injury. This view persisted until the nineteenth century, when Rudolf Virchow, who considered inflammation a pathological condition, added loss of function (*functio laesa*) to the list as the fifth cardinal sign of inflammation.

Today, inflammation is defined as "a complex set of interactions among soluble factors and cells that can arise in any tissue in response to traumatic, infections, post-ischemic, toxic, or autoimmune injury." Certain health conditions will end in the suffix, "-itis," which indicates "inflammation of."

Health Condition	Inflammation of the....
Arthritis	Joints
Bronchitis	Bronchus
Esophagitis	Esophagus
Gastritis	Stomach
Gingivitis	Gums
Meningitis	Brain
Pancreatitis	Pancreas
Rhinitis	Rhinitis
Sinusitis	Sinus

More simply put, inflammation is our body's natural defense to a foreign body, such as a bacteria, toxin, or virus. Once the immune system has completed its job and has destroyed the invader, the body then cools down and returns to a state of equilibrium.

However, if the body is chronically exposed to injury by the food we eat, by alcohol, tobacco, ultraviolet radiation, chronic stress, environmental pollutants, altered gut microbiota, sedentary lifestyle, micronutrient deficiencies, poor diets and improper cooking techniques, inflammation becomes chronic. The human body was never designed to be "chronically" inflamed. Chronic inflammation is as harmful to the body as acute inflammation is helpful.

Usually, when we have an injury outside of the body, like a cut or even a broken bone, we feel and see it. We can most often determine the cause of the injury, and thus the cause of the pain. But what if the occasional discomforts you experience—gastric reflux, joint discomfort, headaches, fatigue, irritable bowel, sinusitis, and even memory loss and brain fog—are also signals of your body crying out in pain from chronic inflammation and injury to the cells. You don't see the insult, but it is there.

Cardiologists can see chronic inflammation of a diseased artery. It has been described as appearing like someone took a stiff brush and scrubbed it repeatedly until it became red, bloody, and infected, just as if that brush were repeatedly rubbed on your hand until it started bleeding, swelling, and eventually become infected. Regardless of whether the inflammatory process occurs internally or externally, if it is chronic, the damage is the same. And the damage occurs in every cell of the body, leading to a multitude of diseases and disorders.

2) **Obesity**:

In addition to the insults that we now know contribute to chronic inflammation and disease in the body, we have recently discovered that adipose tissue (excess body fat) also causes dysfunction that leads to inflammation. Previously, adipose cells were thought to simply be passive depots for energy (storage of excess calories) and nothing more. Now we know the activity of these cells is far from passive. Increased visceral fat (fat surrounding the abdominal organs, i.e. belly fat) releases an abundance of free fatty acids and chemicals like TNF-alpha, adiponectin, resistin, leptin, and other inflammatory substances. This activity promotes and exacerbates insulin resistance and sets up a self-perpetuating cycle that increases insulin resistance. These chemicals result from the instability of the fatty tissue that has increased in size, multiplied in number, and then ruptured, releasing these inflammatory chemicals.

Although obesity *predisposes* one to metabolic dysfunction, there is now evidence to show that obesity is not a determinant of metabolic dysfunction. The presence of type 2 diabetes in the Asian population, who are fairly lean, is evidence of this.

Normally, if there is not an excess of visceral fat in the mitochondria (powerhouse of the cell), the healthy body burns up any free fatty acids that were not needed. But once the obesity sets in, the cascade caused by the chemicals released by the adipose tissue impairs the body's ability to burn fats. This excess fat then spills over into non-fat tissue, like the liver, pancreas, and muscles, and damages them. This is termed lipotoxicity, and it increases insulin resistance and the likely development of type 2 diabetes.

Furthermore, being overweight (not even obese) and inflamed causes leptin resistance. Leptin is a hormone produced by body fat that tells the brain to stop eating when it is full. You don't want to become leptin-resistant because you will continue to eat, and that will perpetuate the problem. Leptin also tells the brain to increase physical activity and increase metabolic rate (all good things that are canceled out when you become leptin-resistant). As fat accumulates, more leptin is released and causes more fat to be burned, but eventually, when too much fat accumulates, the body becomes resistant to the signal of leptin. It doesn't hear it any more. It's like when you are always yelling at your kids to do something. You know they hear you, but they are not listening to you anymore. They have become resistant to your guidance.

As fat cells continue to expand (caused by an influx of too much sugar), they start producing excess reactive oxygen species (ROS). We are exposed every day to ROS in the form of pollutants, smoke, drugs, tobacco, radiation, and xenobiotics (substances foreign to the body). The body also makes its own ROS during normal metabolism and detoxification processes. But when there is excess body fat the body goes into overdrive in the production of ROS. It can't effectively eliminate the excessive amount, and thus more inflammation and toxicity occur.

Obesity itself contributes to inflammation, and this inflammation causes the up-regulation of certain genes involved with the inflammatory response. The immune system tries to reduce the inflammation and the resulting damage while leaving debris (inflammatory by-products) in the process. In essence, the body starts attacking itself. Consequently, we have an emerging epidemic of autoimmune conditions, including rheumatoid arthritis, Hashimoto's thyroiditis, ankylosing spondylitis, multiple sclerosis, and more.

Now you can see that excess belly fat accumulating around the waist is not simply extra weight. It is a metabolically active organ that is killing us through chronic inflammation, leptin resistance, and oxidative stress (e.g.ROS). It is, therefore, setting the stage for metabolic dysfunction, including type 2 diabetes.

3) **Activation of a genetic predisposition:**

There is no question that genetics play a role in contributing to obesity and belly fat (and type 2 diabetes). The study of the effects of the environment on our genes (modification of gene expression rather than alteration of the genetic code) is termed epigenetics. The environment doesn't change the genetic code, but it does modify our genes, and these modified genes can be passed down to at least one successive generation. Above your genome (all the genetic material inside your cells) lingers this epigenetic master plan that determines if your genes get turned on or off and to what degree. So, yes, genes are important, but even more important are the environmental triggers that can lead to the metabolic dysfunction causing disease.

A long list of genes is associated with obesity (and type 2 diabetes), which is beyond the scope of this book to explore. The more of these genes you have, the higher is your risk of developing obesity (and type 2 diabetes). Genetic testing for these genes may be beneficial. Regardless, if you are at an increased risk for disease due to your genetics, remember it is our "modern" lifestyle that will TRIGGER or activate the genes that will develop the disease. Even if you have these bad genes, the condition will remain dormant until activated. You must load the gun for it to fire. For example, evidence suggests that those with a genetic predisposition to type 2 diabetes do not develop type 2 diabetes if they are not exposed to the negative environmental factors. That's good news!

So, to summarize this highly technical discussion, here is a succinct and simple equation that identifies the culprits leading to belly fat:

Modern Lifestyle + Genetic Predisposition = Belly Fat

Although this is a simple equation, now you understand that the cause of obesity and accompanying belly fat involves many complex factors. If it were simple, we wouldn't have an obesity epidemic.

Remember the concerns of the JAMA editors that the food and restaurant industries may be in part responsible? Well, I can assure you that the food industry most definitely understands the complexity of weight gain all too well. They hire scientists who know how the mechanisms in our bodies that work to keep us addicted to their products, and they engineer their food products with the intent to keep us addicted and craving their foods. If you don't believe me, please read the book by Michael Moss called *Salt Sugar Fat: How the Food Giants Hooked Us*. You can learn more at MichaelMossBooks.com.

So, in addition to dealing with a conventional healthcare system designed to keep us sick, we must be aware that the food industry sabotages us. Are you ready to say enough is enough? Your difficulty in losing belly fat has not been totally your fault, so please stop beating yourself up about it. If you have been on countless diets and have lost the weight (as expected) but gained it back plus some, you are a victim. It is not your fault. "Fool me once, but don't fool me twice" should now be your mantra, since you now have the roadmap to find your way to true health—and, of course, wealth.

CHAPTER 5

Minimize Belly Fat

"Health doesn't happen in the doctor's office! It happens in the kitchen, the grocery store, and the community!"
~ Dr. Mark Hyman, Director,
Cleveland Center for Functional Medicine

Finding Your Weigh: Energy Balance

Where to start?

Let me first get something straight before you start reading this next section and think how totally out-of-date I must be. In the next few pages, I will be presenting some facts about "energy balance." You must understand this foundational information to minimize belly fat before going on to the next section. It's not comprehensive; it's just the beginning. I don't want you to start feeling discouraged and hopeless if you have been working unsuccessfully with this concept. You may have just had one piece of the puzzle. Be patient, and I will put the pieces together, as simply as possible.

I have created a belly fat (weight) loss program I call "GET Balanced, Fit, and Slim Step-Power® Transformation." The first step of the way (or "weigh," as I like to say!) to belly fat (weight) loss freedom is to balance your energy.

What is energy?

Just as an automobile uses gasoline or electricity as fuel for energy, all living creatures need fuel to function. Human fuel is food. We measure the energy stored in our foods by measuring calories (kcal). A calorie is simply a measure of energy. If you consume more energy than your body needs, the extra energy will be stored as body fat. This extra energy will be "waisted" (pun intended).

For the purpose of managing weight, there are two very distinct roles of the food we eat. The first is the control of body fat, using the concept of energy balance (calories in and calories out). Most people would have you believe that weight loss is a function of calorie intake. It is, but it is not the complete picture, which I will explain when I discuss the second distinct role of food. For now, let's continue learning more about energy balance.

It's not enough to say any fuel or any food will provide us with the energy we need to run efficiently. When you are shopping for a new automobile, other than the make and model of it, you are also interested in its fuel efficiency, aren't you? How many miles per gallon does it get on the highway? How many miles per gallon does it get when city driving? Fuel efficiency is also important when it comes to fueling the body. The amount of fuel (calories) you require is determined by your gender, height, weight, age, and how well you are performing on the highway or city (for example, are you sedentary or active?).

Formulas can calculate how much fuel you need (your calorie needs) to maintain your current weight. There are also tools called indirect calorimeters that will measure your basal metabolic rate. For those who are having difficulty with weight loss, I highly recommend seeking out a professional who can measure this for you. Otherwise, a calorie calculator, like the one found at Calculator.net/calorie-calculator.html might provide you a decent estimate.

Classifying your degree of overweight or obesity

What is your goal weight? Before answering this question, let's first determine where you stand regarding your degree of overweight or obesity by today's standard recommendations (do take this with a grain of salt). Currently, two standards assess a person's degree of body weight health to determine if their weight is considered normal, overweight, or obese.

The first standard is the Body Mass Index (BMI).

Let's stop here so you can figure out what your BMI is. Go to this website:

Calculator.net/bmi-calculator.html, where you will enter your height, weight, gender, and age for your results. See the chart below for the meaning of your BMI results.

Category	BMI range (kg/m²)
Severe Thinness	<16
Moderate Thinness	16-17
Mild Thinness	17-18.5
Normal	18.5-25
Overweight	25-30
Obese Class I	30-35
Obese Class II	35-40
Obese Class III	>40

The second standard is the Waist Circumference (WC).

Assessing WC is the most practical tool to evaluate abdominal fat before and during weight loss treatment.

A high-risk waist circumference is considered:
>40 inches (102 cm) for men and >35 inches (88 cm) for women

Often, standard charts and formulas used to assess ideal body weight are unrealistic. One reason is because a person's "actual" amount of muscle mass is not taken into consideration in charts and formulas. Scales and calculations based on height cannot assess muscle mass. Just like the best way to assess calorie requirements is with a personalized assessment using an indirect calorimeter, the best way to determine an ideal body weight is a personalized assessment with a body composition analysis. This test will provide you with a close approximation of your muscle mass. When we have this data, we can then calculate your "ideal body weight" based on your muscle mass.

You see, a major goal during weight loss is to make sure that the weight being lost is fat, not muscle. We want to preserve muscle because it is metabolically active and will assist with losing weight.

When people go on diets, they often consume too few calories, losing muscle mass and slowing metabolism. This is not an issue if you are following the guidelines I will share later in this book for protein and other macronutrient recommendations.

When one starts a weight loss program, it would be ideal to have monthly body composition measurements to assess if the weight loss is coming from fat and not muscle. If you are losing muscle during your program, adjustments must be made.

What is your weight goal?

Often, simply losing five to ten percent of body weight will deliver dramatic improvements in your overall health. It may be that you recall a weight you felt good at in the past and you want to return to that weight. If you are unable to have a body composition analysis completed to assess your ideal body weight, you may consider using the easy "Hamwi" method to determine an appropriate weight for you. Here's the calculation:

For males: For your first five feet in height, give yourself 106 pounds. For every inch over five feet, add six pounds. For example, if you are 6'2", your ideal body weight is 190 pounds +/- 10 percent, or a range of 171 to 209 pounds.

For females: For your first five feet in height, give yourself 100 pounds. For every inch over five feet, add five pounds for each additional inch. For example, if you are 5'4", your ideal body weight is 120 pounds +/- 10 percent, or a range of 108-132 pounds.

What is a safe amount of weight loss?

For most people, a safe and realistic weight loss is one-half to two pounds per week. In some circumstances (say, if you are morbidly obese), it might be acceptable to set a larger goal of three pounds per week, but this is best considered on an individual basis. A slow and steady weight loss is safe and realistic. Sure, you can lose more weight than this initially, but fast weight loss is not FAT loss; it is WATER loss, and the weight most always comes right back on. That's not what you want. You want permanent weight loss, and you want to develop healthy eating patterns along the way, without feeling deprived. Please, don't even consider trying to follow one of those fad diets to gain leverage. I promise it will backfire. You will regain the weight you lost and more.

Also, please avoid purchasing food products from popular commercial weight loss programs. One of my clients was eating farm-fresh, non-processed foods and having great results. He thought he could hasten his weight loss by purchasing prepared meals from a well-meaning relative who sold the products. He would continue to work with me, but he wouldn't have to cook his meals. He lost forty pounds in eight weeks! Amazing, right? I was impressed. I couldn't figure out how he was losing so much weight so quickly, since my plan is not designed to result in so much weight loss so fast.

Then we discovered his blood pressure increased from 135/75 to 180/95. I was perplexed. I would have expected a decrease in his blood pressure with a weight loss of forty pounds. I solved the mystery when he told me he was using these prepackaged foods five times a day, not realizing that each contained 390 mg of sodium, for a total of 1950 mg of sodium. The recommended sodium intake per day is 1500 mg. And he was still eating other foods throughout the day. I estimate he was consuming at least three times the recommended sodium intake. His blood work also showed an elevation in his inflammatory markers.

I explained to him the dangers of this. I urged him to stop the meals. But he was impatient, and he wanted a quicker fix. Then he began getting headaches, fatigue, dizziness, and heart palpitations. His doctor added another blood pressure medication, and the fatigue worsened, his libido dropped, and his headaches worsened. He finally agreed to stop the prepackaged meals.

Please know that there are no magical bullets. Admittedly, it takes work. But nothing worthwhile in life comes easy. You can do this. Remember, too, that a positive attitude and a willing spirit go a long way.

Remember: SAFE = PERMANENT = REALISTIC

What should your calorie deficit be?

Every time we consume an extra 3,500 calories, our body will store an extra pound of body fat (according to the First Law of Thermodynamics, which we will talk about later and possibly rebuke). With this mathematical calculation, if we eat an extra one hundred calories a day beyond what our body needs, every single day of the year, we can expect to gain ten pounds by the end of the year.

3500 calories = 1 pound

To Lose One Pound Per Week—> Create a Deficit of 500 Calories Per Day

3500 calories ÷ 7 days per week = 500 calories

To Lose Two Pounds Per Week—> Create a Deficit of 1000 Calories Per Day

7000 calories ÷ 7 days per week = 1000 calories

Sample Plan to Lose One Pound Per Week
(creating a 500 calorie per day deficit):

Reduce your calorie intake by 300 calories per day + Burn an additional 200 calories a day with purposeful physical activity.

Lose weight by eating less than your body burns.

It's really not that hard to cut three hundred calories a day from your usual diet routine. In fact, when you follow all of the recommended guidelines in this book, it will be a breeze, because honestly, you are going to be eating more delicious, quality food than you have been eating. This food will be amazingly filling and appetite satisfying. You will experience no deprivation.

Also, it's not that hard to burn an additional two hundred calories a day with purposeful physical activity. You might find that one day you eat two hundred calories less food, but that you burn three hundred calories by walking three miles that day. You do not necessarily have to be that consistent every day. Obviously, life intervenes! Ideally, you would like to create a deficit EVERY DAY, but at least work to achieve the desired deficit for the WEEK.

Even if you aren't successful burning the desired number of calories each and every week, you will soon learn that despite the mathematical calculation of calories "in" and calories "out," there are many factors that contribute to "energy balance" besides calories and activity. You will learn about these in the upcoming section.

The strongest factor for success is self-esteem: believing you can do it, believing you deserve it, believing you will get it.

Finding Your Weigh: Appetite Control

I wish I had a dollar for every time a client said, "If only I had more willpower, I would not have a weight problem" or for when they asked me for a medication to decrease their appetite. First of all, realize that there is no such thing as willpower. Willpower is nonexistent, and the belief that willpower is necessary for weight loss will always lead to failure. Instead of willpower, what is needed is a "willingness" to consider new ideas and methods such as the ones presented in this book.

I would like you to consider rebuking everything I just told you in this chapter about energy balance (well not everything, exactly). We discussed configuring the correct amount of fuel needed to determine fuel efficiency. We discussed how an automobile's fuel efficiency is determined by its make and model, which is affected by its driving conditions (city or highway driving). The amount of energy the body requires to function is also dependent on similar conditions (our make/model and movement conditions).

Also, I mentioned the concept of the First Law of Thermodynamics. You can't argue with the First Law of Thermodynamics that says that the regulation of body weight is dependent on the maintenance of energy balance.

According to this law, energy can neither be created nor destroyed but can be inter-converted between different forms. The human body is a chemical device that takes in chemical energy (food) and converts it into other forms of energy (stored compounds) and into mechanical work and heat. Here is the formula:

Energy intake (food) = Energy expended (heat, work, biosynthesis)
+ Energy stored

Imbalance in this equation results in a change in body weight. If the energy intake is greater than the energy expended, the excess energy must be stored (in the form of body fat) and if energy expenditure exceeds that of energy intake, a decrease in body weight occurs.

> *Because of the First Law of Thermodynamics, this occurs with absolute certainty.*

Are all calories the same?

We cannot argue with the First Law of Thermodynamics. Or can we? Actually, we can! You see, the First Law of Thermodynamics says that energy is conserved in a system, which means a *closed* system. So, for example, if I were to take one thousand calories of soda and one thousand calories of broccoli and burn them in a laboratory, the same amount of energy will be released from each. That is FACT!

The problem is that our body is NOT a closed system. The body's metabolism depends on more than the amount of fuel. The body's metabolism also depends on the type of fuel that is consumed. Isn't this also similar to the efficiency of an automobile?

Regular gasoline may efficiently run an automobile that requires premium gasoline. And the grade of gasoline will hardly matter if the proper amount and type of oil are not present, which will ultimately also affect fuel efficiency. What if there is an oil leak? That would certainly affect fuel efficiency, right?

In the body, water serves as the lubricant that oil serves in a car. The body systems require adequate and clean water for lubrication and efficient maintenance. In addition to the water we drink, we also get water from our foods (if we are consuming the proper ones). If we are consuming water in the form of sodas, coffee, etc., we may have a water leak, because these beverages are considered to be diuretics and cause us to lose nutrients that are needed for metabolism and improved fuel efficiency.

Bottom line: Fuel type matters!

The problem with a thousand calories of soda is that it might give us temporary energy, but it is also going to turn all types of hormonal signals on in the body that drive weight gain and cause inflammation (which hinders weight loss). Soda causes triglycerides to increase, good HDL cholesterol to decrease, testosterone to decrease, appetite to increase, an increased risk of fatty liver, and it is void of any type of micronutrients to aid in metabolism. Soda causes shifts in the body's fat-burning ability and leads to an inflammatory mess that will not allow the body to let go of the fat.

On the other hand, if you eat a thousand calories of broccoli (hypothetically, of course), the exact opposite happens. Your appetite decreases, and you get full because of its high fiber content. It is very low in sugar, therefore, it will reduce the risk of inflammation. Its nutrient content supports detoxification of the liver (rather than the promotion of fatty liver) and aids in an overall increase in metabolism. So, these examples rebuke the First Law of Thermodynamics. Eating the same amount of calories from different foods will not result in the same amount of weight loss. In fact, weight gain is likely to occur when eating the wrong type of foods, even if calorie intake is reduced. Therefore, the answer is NO...all calories are NOT the same.

Appetite

The first distinct role of food is the control of body fat, using the concept of energy balance (calories in and calories out). Although this is a big part of managing weight, it is not the complete picture.

The second distinct role food plays in weight management is appetite control. Appetite is not the same as hunger. Appetite, the desire to satisfy both the physiological need for food and to experience the pleasure from food, is controlled by signals in our brain. Can we control these signals, and therefore our appetite? Absolutely! And I don't mean with weight loss medications. The appetite is controlled by many factors, mostly from the foods we consume. The wrong foods don't give the body the information it requires to heal itself and properly function, and that includes allowing it to achieve an ideal body weight.

Like everything in the body, food provides nutrients that bathe every living cell, including the cells that control your appetite. Appetite correlates to chemicals manufactured within the brain cells, which are manufactured from the foods in the diet. If you want to better control the impulses that control your appetite, you have to learn how and when to eat the proper foods. So, you see, although calorie intake is hugely important in weight management, the foods you choose have more significance than calorie intake alone. Hence, consuming a well-balanced diet that includes fruits, vegetables, protein, and fiber, and minimizing (preferably eliminating) processed & poorly prepared foods is the best way to control your appetite.

Attitude is everything

> A negative attitude is like a flat tire.... You can't go anywhere
> until you change it.
>
> ~ Author Unknown

Some of the chemicals affecting appetite can also affect your mood. Your diet can change your attitude about eating and the way you feel about yourself. The right attitude about trying new things is very important for weight maintenance. The brain chemicals that control appetite (and mood) respond to lifestyle, behavioral, and environmental changes.

The hardest thing, of course, about decreasing your appetite and choosing the foods that will help change your attitude about eating, that will ultimately lead to belly fat loss, is getting started. You may not even want to take the first step because you are not yet programmed with the right attitude, because you are not yet programmed with the right diet. It's like the "chicken and the egg," scenario. Which came first, the chicken or the egg?

Bottom line: There are some things in life that we just have to do, whether we like to do them or not. If you don't do something now to begin living a healthier life, you will be paying for it years later. You may then be faced with weekly trips to your healthcare provider, taking pharmaceutical medications that may cause side effects, missing quality time with your family because you are too weak, too tired, or in too much pain to participate, and so on.

Note: This section about appetite control was significantly simplified. I have not discussed the scientific data of the effects of hormones on satiety and appetite signals due to space limitations.

Finding Your Weigh: Defining Your Wellness Vision

What is your wellness vision?

You have heard the saying before: "If you don't know where you are going, any road will get you there."

First, you must develop your "wellness vision" to get on the road to improving your health!

If your wellness vision is to "lose weight," you are on the wrong road, and you will likely not get to your destination.

What is wellness?

Wellness is not simply the opposite of illness. It is so much more than that. Wellness has been defined as:

* a condition of good physical and mental health
* the mastery of one's well being that includes the regular practice of physical, mental, emotional, and spiritual behaviors
* a way of life that encompasses nutritional, physical, stress management, and health maintenance, or disease prevention strategies

Wellness doesn't happen naturally. We need to plan and take action to improve or maintain wellness. The society we live in makes achieving wellness much more difficult, but not impossible. Anything in life worth having, not just health, is worth working toward. You'll need a vision for what you want in life.

What is a wellness vision?

A wellness vision is the motivating factor, the "why" you desire to lose weight. The "why" is your road map that will get you to your destination.

BEGIN with the END in mind.

There are no right or wrong wellness visions. But you must have one. The goal of "losing weight" is not enough. Of course, you want to lose weight, but you first must have a good reason.

What a wellness vision can do

A wellness vision can define behaviors you want to incorporate, such as getting regular exercise, or to eat more vegetables, or to get more sleep. A wellness vision can define outcomes you want to achieve, including weight loss, a lower cholesterol level, greater strength and fitness, and less stress. A wellness vision can define motivators you want to experience: feeling better, looking younger, feeling energetic, appearing less tired. These ultimately will also have a positive effect on your goal for belly fat loss.

The wellness vision can also include obstacles you want to overcome, such as eating poorly when you are stressed, skipping exercise when you are tired, not cooking healthy meals when you are too busy. The wellness vision also can reveal strategies that will help you overcome the obstacles, like purchasing pre-cut or pre-washed vegetables to reduce meal preparation time and splitting up your exercise time into three ten-minute sessions instead of one thirty-minute session.

What is your wellness vision?

Sure, you already know the many reasons why excess belly fat is unhealthy, but that still might not matter to you. That might not be a strong enough motivator to lose weight. Is there a deeper, more powerful reason you want to lose weight? You need to figure out what this is for you. In other words, you need to know "why" you are trying to approach a healthy weight and determine if this reason is important enough for you to make the changes you will need to make. Because as humans, let's face it: we don't do anything we don't want to do. But, by golly, we always do what we want to do. We complain that we don't have time to exercise, or we don't have time to cook a decent meal, but somehow we manage to find the time to play a round of golf or get our nails done or smoke a cigarette or go to a movie or go out to dinner, or whatever it is that is important to us.

Simple ways to motivate yourself every day:

- Have a clear vision. Review the principles above.
- Get passionate about your vision. Do whatever you have to do to fuel this passion and stay on course.
- Work hard to get results. The harder you work, the better the results, and the better the results you get, the more you will be motivated to get more.
- Nourish your mind. Read books that teach you new ideas and skills, read stories of successful people, listen to motivational tapes. Listening and learning about other people's success is a powerful motivator for your own success.
- Ride the wave of momentum. Take it when it comes. When you feel good about your successes, take advantage of it, and get as much out of it as you can.
- Stay committed to the course. Know what you stand for. When you are presented with challenges that would lead to

the opposite outcome you are seeking (and you will be), your commitment will offer no doubt or hesitation in your choice. If you are committed to living a Christian life, you won't consider shoplifting, even if an easy opportunity presented itself. The same applies to the commitment of leading a healthy life. If you are offered a Krispy Kreme donut, and you are deeply committed, you would never accept it because of the negative impact it will have on your body.

Examples of wellness visions:

- My wellness vision for the next three months is to reverse my recent trend of weight gain so I can look better in my clothes, feel younger, and have more energy to play with my kids.
- My wellness vision for the next year is to reduce my stress, so I can begin to cook meals instead of eating out in restaurants.
- My wellness vision is to lose ten pounds and to maintain this loss so I can look good in my bikini on my fortieth birthday.
- My wellness vision is to increase my strength and stamina, so I can remain self-sufficient without the aid of outside assistance, and to have the energy to play with my grandchildren.
- My wellness vision in the next two years is to achieve a healthy weight and prevent my pre-diabetes from turning into diabetes.
- My wellness vision in the next six months is to establish a routine exercise program to delay the aging process and preserve my ability to perform the activities of daily living in my senior years, independently.
- My wellness vision in the next year is to improve my cholesterol level to reduce my risk of heart disease.
- My wellness vision is to establish healthy eating habits, so I can be a good role model to my children and grandchildren.
- My wellness vision is to take charge of my health and achieve a greater sense of well-being and contentment.

If you don't write down your vision and your goals, they are only ideas. Writing down your goals and your vision significantly improve your chances of success. Take your ideas to reality by writing them down.

CHAPTER 6

Feed the Belly

"Real food doesn't have ingredients. Real food is ingredients."
~ Jamie Oliver, Celebrity Chef

How you eat and what you eat can help you avoid the need for pharmaceutical medications, keep you out of doctors' offices, and help you live life to the fullest. My nine fundamental principles for feeding the belly are not principles of "dieting," but principles for living a balanced and healthy life.

1) **Plan to Succeed**:

Benjamin Franklin said it best, *"If you fail to plan, you plan to fail."*

Here's the thing: Humans start feeling hunger about every three to five hours. We can count on this. The length of time between meals may change, depending on the quality of the diet. If hunger is not satisfied, discomfort increases, and you will consume whatever is in sight. Often, this means consuming the completely wrong things. Often, these completely wrong things lead to cravings for more of the wrong things. You eventually find yourself in a vicious cycle of feeding the body unhealthy food because you have failed to plan.

Solution: Be prepared before those hunger pangs occur, and be armed with the appropriate fuel. When you fuel your body and mind with the right foods, you will find the hunger pangs will be less painful, you will be able to go longer periods between eating, you will be more satisfied, and you will prevent the erratic highs and lows of blood sugar excursions.

Planning means "doing your research to locate the grocery stores and their aisles that will have the purest and healthiest foods." (See Appendix 1 for Clean Food Resources.) Initially, plan on having all the items you need for a one-week menu. You may even need to plan to prepare meals in advance for the week.

Planning also means reviewing your menus for tomorrow and possibly putting your lunch and breakfast items together the night before.

Planning means always carrying a safe snack with you to have when you are unable to eat your next meal as planned. And of course, planning means understanding exactly what "safe" snacks and foods are, which will require you to continue enlightening yourself through the pages of this book.

Planning is the KEY to your success in any endeavor, especially one involving feeding your belly.

2) **Eat Organic** (and avoid foods with labels):

If you do nothing else, try to make it a priority to purchase "clean" food. "Clean" food has not been exposed to harmful chemicals (toxins). As you know, the chemicals the body cannot recognize and that consequently disrupt its metabolic processes contribute to inflammation and overall health risks that lead to the use of pharmaceutical medications. So, "eating clean" means ditching the processed foods and getting back to the basics---real food. Is this always easy to do? Obviously, not, in our modern society, but remember, our "modern" lifestyle has led to our use of pharmaceutical medications. For more clarity on what it means to eat clean, refer to Appendix 2 for a Guide to Eating Whole Foods and to Appendix 3 for a Guide on Food Quality that will explain the various food labeling on meat, eggs, and dairy.

PRESCRIPTION DETOX | 85

Why Should You Eat Organic?

Remember: Food is information. Food with the right information gives your body what it needs and craves, and it will allow your body to heal itself without pharmaceutical medications. If the food is adulterated with chemicals, your body will get confused and unable to properly process the nutrients in that food because it is too busy trying to detoxify and eliminate the foreign components (unrecognizable food additives and pesticides).

One of the biggest obstacles I hear to eating clean is that it is too expensive. I am going to bust this belief: what is expensive is buying fake and contaminated food that your body doesn't need and eating it. Then you find yourself going back and forth to doctors' offices, missing work, burning automotive gasoline, shelling out office co-pays, and purchasing needless "Band-Aid" prescriptions. Can you afford that expense and hassle, not to mention the long-lasting negative consequences to your body?

If you are trying to cut corners on your food budget, instead of cutting out organically grown food, consider instead eliminating processed foods. A significant expense and waste are associated with most processed foods. Think about the packaging costs associated with processed foods, not to mention the health risks from the addition of artificial flavor enhancers, trans fats, hydrogenated oils, chemical colors and preservatives, excessive sodium, white flour, and sugar that wreak havoc on your health. These risks jeopardize your personal health, resulting in chronic diseases that burden the healthcare system and lead to people taking over ten prescription medications at once. When you cut out processed foods and concentrate on purchasing wholesome organic food, you will reap the benefits of improved health, and it will become obvious to you that buying organic is money well spent.

To save money when purchasing organic foods, shop locally, look for bargains, and shop when items are in season since the cost will be lower when there is a greater supply. Consider joining a food co-op, and purchase generic organic products versus name brands to save on organic food costs. (See Appendix 1 for further resources.)

In addition to reducing your exposure to harmful pesticides, eating organically may also reduce your exposure to hormones, antibiotics, and potentially harmful irradiated food. Less antibiotic use may help to avoid the development of antibiotic resistance. Organic beef, chicken, and poultry are raised on 100 percent organic feed and never given antibiotics or hormones. Also, their meat is never irradiated. Organic milk and eggs come from animals not given antibiotics or hormones and fed 100 percent organic feed for the previous twelve months. (Free-range eggs come from hens that are allowed to roam, but they are not guaranteed to be organic.)

According to The Institute for Functional Medicine (IFM), several studies support the claim that organic diets can dramatically reduce pesticide exposure. One such study compared pesticide metabolite levels in eighteen children who got at least 75 percent of their juice and produce servings from organic sources with those in twenty-one children who got at least 75 percent of their juice and produce from conventionally grown food. Levels of organophosphorus pesticide metabolites in the urine collected were six to nine times higher in the children who ate conventionally grown foods than in those who ate organic diets. Other studies have corroborated these claims.

Claims of enhanced nutritional benefits of organic foods have caused much controversy. However, studies have been able to support this claim. The *Journal of Alternative and Complementary Medicine* reported one study showing that, on average, organic crops contain 86 percent more chromium, 29 percent more magnesium, 27 percent more vitamin C, 21 percent more iron, 26 percent more calcium, 42 percent more manganese, 498 percent more iodine, and 372 percent more selenium. Significantly fewer nitrates also were found in the organic food. Nitrogen-based fertilizers can elevate nitrates in food and drinking water, which can be converted to potentially carcinogenic nitrosamines.

What foods are most important to eat organically?

Organic meats and dairy appear to be the most heavily contaminated with hormones, pesticides, and herbicides. According to a 2009 study that was a joint effort between the United States Department of Agriculture (USDA) and researchers at Clemson University in South Carolina, grass-fed beef is better for human health than grain-fed beef in these top ten ways:

- Lower in total fat
- Higher in beta-carotene
- Higher in vitamin E (alpha-tocopherol)
- Higher in the B-vitamins thiamin and riboflavin
- Higher in the minerals calcium, magnesium, and potassium
- Higher in total omega-3s
- Better ratio of omega-6 to 3 fatty acids
- Higher in CLA (conjugated linoleic acid), a potential cancer fighter
- Higher in vaccenic acid (which can be transformed into CLA)
- Lower in the saturated fats linked with heart disease

Produce can be quite variable. If you are unable to eat organic produce, it is wise to be aware of those products that are the least contaminated with pesticides. The Environmental Working Group (EWG) publishes two lists, "Dirty Dozen" and "Clean Fifteen," that are updated annually. (See Appendix 1 for internet links.)

To determine if the produce you are purchasing at the supermarket is organic, check the PLU (product look-up) code on the produce sticker. If the number code is simply four digits, the produce is conventionally grown. If the PLU code is a five-digit code beginning with a "9" the product is organic (and not genetically-modified). The prefix "8" was built into the code standard to identify genetically-modified organisms (GMOs), but unfortunately because using PLU codes is voluntary, it was never used, therefore, you cannot identify GMOs in this way. Thus, conventionally grown produce could be genetically-modified.

Eating clean and organic also means avoiding foods with labels. We generally think of labels as good, helping us assess the contents of the food product. Well, yes, this is true. But it is commonly the labeled foods that are highly processed. You don't find fruits and vegetables with labels on them (except for the coding discussed above). Continue to read the labels of the food products that you purchase, but only purchase them if the ingredient label has no more than five ingredients. If you cannot pronounce the ingredient or know what that ingredient is, put it back on the shelf, not in your grocery cart. Refer to Appendix 1 for online farms and companies to purchase your organic meats, seafood, snacks, and other clean products.

3) **Eat More Carbs**—Non-starchy vegetable carbs, that is:

Americans are carb-oholics, and we come by it naturally. The food industry has sabotaged our taste buds. Food scientists working for the food industry know exactly how to get us addicted to their products. It's no accident you crave carbohydrates—it's by design.

Eating the wrong type and amount of carbohydrates is the root cause of many health conditions, including diabetes and cancer. Unfortunately, Americans have been misled for far too long, thanks to the USDA Food Pyramid, which recommended that 50 percent of calories come from carbohydrates. The body does not need this much carbohydrate. In addition, because of another misguided diet recommendations to eat low-fat, additional sugar and salt have been added to our foods to make up for the fat that was removed. Good grief! Talk about a total debacle in trusting our government to provide us with nutrition guidelines that were totally bogus and incorrect, and consequently contributed to our nation's healthcare dilemma. Hello! We need healthy fat in our diets, not additional sugar and salt.

Sugar is the enemy, and if you are not yet aware of it, all carbohydrates breakdown into sugar! Two slices of bread contain approximately thirty grams of carbohydrate, which breaks down to be almost as much sugar as in a twelve-ounce can of cola.

Did you know that sugar is as addictive as cocaine? It excites the same brain neurons as does cocaine, and the more you eat it, the more you want.

Did you know that cancer is a sugar-feeder? Cancer is an obligate glucose-metabolizer, which means it has an obligation to consume sugar to survive.

Sugar weakens the innate immune system and leaves the body open to all types of health conditions including common chronic complaints, such as headaches, joint pain, lack of energy, poor sleep, and of course, diabetes. When sugar is removed from the diet for two to three weeks, many of these long-standing complaints just disappear.

Today, it's not easy to avoid sugar since it is in so many food products, including spaghetti sauce, salad dressings, crackers, breads, and canned soups (another reason to avoid processed foods). The good news is if you just give yourself a chance to get sugar out of your system, you won't miss it.

Before you start hating me for taking away all your favorite foods, let me explain that there are ways "to have your cake and eat it too!" I love cake, pies, and cookies just like the next guy, but they are not a staple in my diet. If I choose to eat them, I do it with a plan in mind, replacing a starchy vegetable or fruit. Honestly, though, if I am eating healthy most of the time and giving my body what it needs, I rarely crave these types of foods. My plan replaces the high-carbohydrate food items with low carbohydrate alternatives: almond flour in place of white flour, mashed cauliflower in place of mashed potatoes, cauliflower pizza crust, and cauliflower tortillas. Other grain-free alternatives include shirataki noodles, cauliflower rice, flax seed crackers, and zucchini noodles. Search online for recipes for these ideas. You can also go to my website for meal/food ideas. See the link in Appendix 4.

Another plan to reduce my desire for carbohydrates is to be sure I include enough healthy fats in my diet. Eating the right foods in the right amounts will prevent the carbohydrate cravings.

Fruit is also a carbohydrate. Yes, we think of fruit as being a healthy food, and it is, but we tend to eat too much of it. Fruit has some awesome antioxidants, fiber, and vitamins and minerals, so we want to have them in our diet, but in moderation, since they break down into sugar. When eating fruit, it's always best to eat the whole fruit instead of drinking the juice, since the liquid form raises blood sugar—and it raises it very quickly, just as a soda would. The best fruits to eat are berries. If you are making smoothies, only add ½ cup serving. I see so many people thinking they are doing good by having a smoothie, but they add in a whole banana (approximately thirty grams of carbohydrates), 3/4 cup strawberries (around fifteen grams of carbohydrate), plus a cup of juice (thirty grams of carbo-hydrates). OUCH!!!! That's an entire day's worth of carbohydrates and death by sugar.

Fruit sugar is known as fructose. White table sugar is composed of two sugars: glucose and fructose. Glucose is important for the body as long as it is consumed in moderation, but fructose is a different story. Even worse than fructose, however, is high-fructose corn syrup (HFCS). Avoid the consumption of products made with HFCS at all cost. Fructose is not rapidly absorbed into the blood-stream and taken up by the cells like glucose is. Instead, fructose is shunted to the liver, where it is converted to fat. Non-alcoholic fatty liver disease (NAFLD), which is directly linked to diabetes and obesity, is caused by excess fructose consumption.

Milk also contains lactose (milk sugar). People drink a lot of milk, and they think it is good for them. Milk is one of the most common food allergies leading to gastrointestinal problems. I don't recommend most milk products, because of this and because of its sugar content. Instead, I recommend the use of nut milks, which have minimal sugar and are high in healthy fats.

Breakfast cereal is the least healthy make-believe "health" food on the planet. It's unbelievable that it is such a staple in our society. You might as well sit down to a bowl of pure sugar. The fruit we add to the cereal breaks down into sugar, the milk we add to it is composed of sugar, and there is sugar added to the sugar (the cereal itself). I encourage you to eat breakfast, but you are better off skipping it if you are planning a breakfast of this sort. Pancakes or waffles with syrup, oatmeal (yes, I said oatmeal), toast and jam, bagels, donuts, and a tortilla are just as evil. But there are ways to significantly reduce the harmful carbohydrates in these meals. (Refer to Appendix 4 for some recommended low-carbohydrate recipes and websites.)

Cereal and other carb-heavy breakfast foods are made from grain. Here is yet another well-held false belief that grains are healthy. Major cereal grains, like wheat, corn, rice, barley, sorghum, oats, rye and millet, have been the staple crops of the "Standard American Diet" (SAD) and the "poster children" for health organizations like the American Diabetes Association and the American Heart Association, not to mention the endorsement of breakfast cereal companies that advertise their product as the "Breakfast of Champions."

Not only does the body convert grains into sugar. But plants like cereal grains produce toxins, too. They need to protect themselves from predators for survival. Unlike animals that can run away when they are threatened, cereal plants have had to evolve with other mechanisms of protection. Here's how these plants protect themselves:

*   They produce toxins that damage the lining of our gut.
*   They produce toxins that bind essential minerals, making them unavailable to us.
*   They produce toxins that inhibit digestion and absorption of other essential nutrients.

One of the major toxic compounds in cereal grains is the protein gluten. Gluten damages the intestines and makes it leaky. Leaky gut is a serious problem and predisposes one to autoimmune conditions. One does not have to have celiac disease to have an intolerance to gluten. Wheat gluten triggers an immune response in everyone (even if they don't know it) and leads to gut inflammation and auto-immune conditions. This is another major reason to avoid whole grains. (See Appendix 5 for a Guide to Gluten.)

By now you are probably asking yourself, "so how many grams of carbohydrates should I be eating per day?" Historically, we have been counseling people with diabetes to consume approximately fifty percent of their calories from carbohydrates. Well, how is that working for us? In 2012, there were 29.1 million Americans with diabetes. As previously discussed, by the year 2050, it is predicted that one out of three Americans will have diabetes. One reason we have been so liberal is because of the pharmaceutical medications that are prescribed to counteract the excessive intake of carbohydrates that we are giving. How crazy is that? We can no longer afford to be this liberal with carbohydrates and mask the damage they are doing with drugs, not just for people with diabetes, but for most all of us (if we want to avoid disease). Instead, our actual complex carbohydrate needs should only be about twenty percent of our calorie needs. Notice, I am not giving a set amount of carbohydrates, because everyone has different calorie requirements.

As discussed in Chapter 5, once you know your calorie requirements, based on your gender, age, height, weight and activity level (minus a deficit if trying to lose weight), then take twenty percent of that to get the amount of calories from carbohydrates you should consume. Then you take that number and divide it by four (4 calories per gram of carbohydrate), to get the amount of recommended carbohydrate grams you need to consume each day. Keep in mind these are all estimates. See the table below for the grams of carbohydrates you will need based on your approximate calorie needs:

Daily Carbohydrate Needs Based on 20% of Caloric Requirements	
If your calorie requirements are:	Keep your daily carbohydrate intake to:
3000	150 grams
2800	140 grams
2500	125 grams
2200	110 grams
2000	100 grams
1800	90 grams
1600	80 grams
1500	75 grams
1200	60 grams

So now that I have taken away everything you live for, let me take away something else: *artificial sweeteners*. Artificial sweeteners are toxic and help to destroy our gut microbiota (the unique collection of gut flora that inhabits our intestines and influences our immunity, mental health, detoxification, and hormones). We need good gut bacteria to help protect us from many health ailments, while also helping us maintain a healthy weight. Artificial sweeteners contribute to a gut microbiome that promotes weight gain.

Caution: you need to be a detective when reading the ingredient labels on all food products. Ingredients are listed by weight in descending order. (See Appendix 6 for the various names of different sweeteners.) Sweeteners should never be one of the first ingredients on a label (unless it is the product itself, such as stevia). Sweeteners should be listed toward the end of the list of ingredients; if they are at the beginning of the list, avoid that food.

Clearly, you need to be careful in choosing your carbohydrate sources. The body needs carbohydrates, but we want to get them from non-starchy vegetables (like broccoli, spinach, kale, green beans, squash, and carrots) and only a moderate fruit intake. You should minimize your intake of starchy vegetables like potatoes, corn, beans, and peas, and limit grains like bread, rice, pasta, and cereals, since all of these foods break down into sugar. It goes without saying that you need to avoid pastries, sodas, candy, flour, cookies, cakes, etc. Eating this way might take a little planning and education on how to make substitutions, but it is doable and so worth it to get off of pharmaceutical medications and live a healthy life.

4) **Eat High Fiber**:

Fiber is crucial for good health, prevention of cancer, reducing inflammation and blood sugar, and for weight control. Getting adequate fiber allows for daily bowel movements to help us rid the body of harmful toxins. Fiber keeps you full and your appetite better controlled; it also assists with improving cholesterol levels and blood pressure. Get at least thirty-five grams of fiber per day. On average, fruits and vegetables have two to three grams of fiber per serving. One tablespoon of chia seeds has 5.5 grams, while a tablespoon of flax seed has two grams.

Most of your fiber should come from fruits and vegetables and from recommended nutraceuticals (like flax seed and chia seed). Avoiding whole grains does make getting adequate fiber intake a little harder, but just a little, because you will be eating lots of vegetables to make up for the whole grains you are not eating. If your meal plan is not keeping your appetite at bay between meals and/or you are not moving your bowels daily, you may require additional fiber-based appetite suppressants or additional fiber powder. Always drink additional water when increasing your fiber intake.

5) **Eat High-Fat and the Right Fat**:

Be liberal with fat. There is no need to be afraid of fat. Conventional medicine got it all wrong again. Just because fat has more calories per gram than carbohydrate or protein (nine calories per gram for fat verses four calories per gram for both carbohydrate and protein), we have been taught to be afraid of all those additional calories. Not so! In fact, that is the best part about fat. We need to embrace its high-calorie content because it provides us with satiety and keeps us feeling full and satisfied, so we are not craving the wrong foods.

Consumption of healthy fats will not make you fat. But eating fat combined with refined carbohydrates, eating unhealthy fats such as trans and partially hydrogenated fats, and overeating will raise blood sugar, stimulate insulin resistance, increase triglycerides and cholesterol, and make you fat.

Fat is the only macronutrient that has little to no impact on blood sugar and insulin release. It serves as a buffer for the protein and carbohydrates in your diet, slowing the absorption of glucose and amino acids and helping your body regulate sugar levels. If you do this right, healthy fats will make up fifty-five to seventy percent of your total calorie intake (You read that correctly!). This is a far cry from previous government recommendations of less than thirty percent of our calories should come from fats (Again, see where this has gotten us: ranking 29th in the world for life expectancy and 75% of physician office visits resulting in the use of pharmaceutical medications, which are the third leading cause of death!). See the table below for what this looks like in fat grams based on your calorie requirements:

Daily Fat Needs Based on 65% of Caloric Requirements	
If your calorie requirements are:	Consume this amount of fat per day:
3000	216 grams
2800	202 grams
2500	180 grams
2200	159 grams
2000	144 grams
1800	130 grams
1600	115 grams
1500	108 grams
1200	87 grams

When you eat adequate fats, you will not have premature hunger or desire to snack before mealtime. Because fat is a slow-burning fuel, it allows you to keep going without suffering the dramatic energy crashes associated with sugar. Plus, the food cravings disappear once you have regained your ability to burn fat for fuel. (See Appendix 7 for Guide to Fats & Oils and Appendix 8 for Guide to Cooking with Fats & Oils to reduce their oxidation and ability to cause inflammation).

I must caution you, however, on what types of fats you must eliminate from your diet.

a) Industrial fats that are high in omega-6 fatty acids need to be avoided. Industrial fats are vegetable oils like corn, cottonseed, soybean, safflower, sunflower, canola, etc. I bet you thought I was going to say things like butter, lard, and other saturated fats. Nope. I have no problem with you eating these saturated fats. In fact, I encourage you to. The use of these vegetable oils, however, is another example of misguidance by the American Heart Association and American Diabetes Association. These omega-6 oils have been shown to cause inflammation, insulin resistance, and impaired leptin signaling, all of which have been shown to contribute to diabetes and heart disease. (Again, see Appendix 7 and 8)

If you are eating out, especially at fast-food restaurants, you are most definitely being exposed to industrial fats from your foods. Have you ever walked into a McDonald's, a Burger King, or a fried chicken joint and noticed how cloudy the place is? The ongoing oxidation of the oil in the fryers liberates harmful reactive oxygen species into the air. Can you imagine how these oils are oxidizing your insides, basically causing your cells to become rancid? Oxidation is a bad thing and will lead to disease. This is why we need to eat foods that contain antioxidants (wholesome fruits, vegetables, spices, etc.) that will help reduce the natural oxidation caused by metabolism waste products and poor food choices.

b) Partially hydrogenated oils absolutely must be avoided. These are dangerous oils that the Food and Drug Administration (FDA) has advised all food producers and restaurants to remove by June 2018. These oils are formed by taking a vegetable oil, putting it in a tank, pressurizing it, adding nickel, and then forcing some hydrogen atoms to merge with the oil. (Who thinks of doing these things?) You may have heard of this type of oil, called trans fat, vegetable fat, vegetable shortening, and margarine. These fats are semi-solid and have an increased risk of causing cardiovascular disease, as they raise the low-density lipoproteins (LDL) (considered bad cholesterol) and lower high-density lipoproteins (HDL) (considered good cholesterol). These fats are found in processed foods, although many companies have been removing them in preparation for the FDA mandate.

Unfortunately, however, some companies are adding *fully* hydrogenated oils into their ingredients, and for some reason, this is not a problem for the FDA, which is baffling. Fully hydrogenated oils, which are completely solid fats, occur when hydrogens have been added to the liquid oil and then mixed with a vegetable oil and interesterified (chemically altered). Interesterification creates butter-like products from liquid vegetable oils. Unfortunately, interesterified oils have been shown to significantly raise the blood glucose level, making them a poor choice for people with diabetes or on the verge of developing diabetes. So, do you see why it's important just to avoid processed foods altogether? I don't know about you, but I am sick of trusting my health to these food companies who are using us as human guinea pigs and couldn't care less about their customers over their corporate bottom lines.

Healthy fats include monounsaturated fat, omega-3s, and medium chain fatty acids. These types of fats are important for cell membrane health and repair, and they stimulate fat burning. Healthy fats are needed to absorb other micronutrients in our foods and to make hormones. Saturated fats also are safe to consume. Here is more information about the good fats:

a) We were told for years to avoid saturated fats, the long-chain fatty acids found in animal products, such as meat, poultry, and dairy (especially cheese), as well as those found in foods like processed desserts, coconut oil, palm oil, and potato/corn/other chips. Nuts also can contain saturated fats, but much less than these other foods. Recently, saturated fats were cleared of contributing to cardiovascular disease. I am fine with you eating saturated fats, however, please assure that the foods that contain them are organic and of top quality. You don't want to eat the saturated fat on a steak from grain-fed cattle due to the poor-quality diet that was fed to that animal and the toxins that are contained within that fat.

However, go ahead and eat the fat from a grass-fed animal, as there is no problem with that.

b) Omega-3 fats are easily the most deficient nutrient in the modern Western diet. Insufficient intake of these vital and essential dietary components is linked to virtually every modern disease process, weight problems, learning disabilities, and affective disorders. Omega-3 fatty acids are long-chain oils associated with reducing insulin resistance and lipids. They are anti-inflammatory, they elevate mood, and they are a natural anti-depressant and anti-anxiety agent. This is a very important oil to consume daily. Foods high in omega 3-fatty acids are leafy greens, walnuts, walnut oils, oily fish, omega-3 eggs, grass-fed and finished meat and poultry, pasture-fed dairy, flax seeds and oil, and chia seeds. Most people are not able to consume enough omega-3 fatty acids, so fish oil supplements are highly recommended. Of course, lab testing first is always a good thing to have done before any supplementation (see Chapter 8).

c) Medium chain triglycerides (MCT) are fatty acids with only six to ten carbon chains. MCT oils are absorbed easily from the intestines and go directly to the liver, where they are broken down into ketone bodies and effectively burned. (Don't confuse this to ketoacidosis, a complication of very highly elevated blood sugars.) Ketone bodies help regulate glucose, reduce hypoglycemia episodes, facilitate weight loss, and fight against dementia and Alzheimer's. They also enhance athletic performance and improve insulin resistance. MCTs are not stored in fat cells as other types of fats are.

Contrary to what many believe, coconut oil is not the best source of MCTs, as only 10 to 15 percent of coconut oil is MCT. Mammalian milk (human, cow, goat, sheep, and horse) deliver higher ratios of MCTs. MCTs can create intestinal discomfort if overdosed, including diarrhea, so slowly increase the dose to a maximum of one to three tablespoons a day for adults. Children should have lower doses.

Traditionally, frying foods has received a bad rap. However, I hope you now realize that if you are frying your foods in the proper type of oils at the proper smoke point and not using the oil over and over again, this is just fine. It's only when the oil is heated to too high a temperature for that type of oil and the oil is repeatedly used (like in a fast-food restaurant) that you will have significant oxidation products build up. This is what is harmful. So, go ahead and enjoy your fried chicken or fried eggplant cooked at home using fresh coconut oil or lard, beef, or duck fat.

6) **Eat the Right Amount of Protein**:

Protein, critical for growth and cell repair, also promotes a healthy weight and improves detoxification pathways when eaten in the proper amount. Protein suppresses the "hunger" hormone, ghrelin, and increases glucagon levels, which causes us to burn fat. We want the body to be a fat-burning machine so we can maintain a healthy weight and avoid illness. Protein also regulates blood glucose to help delay blood sugar surges when carbohydrates are consumed; therefore, eating protein with a carbohydrate source is important.

However, too much protein per day or meal will be converted to sugar and stored as fat, especially in people who are insulin-resistant (unable to use their insulin properly, thereby leading to elevated blood sugar). Excess protein is also insulinemic, which further aggravates insulin resistance.

A fine line marks the correct amount of protein. Typically, protein needs range from 10 to 20 percent of calorie requirements, but studies have shown that a diet with 15 percent of calories coming from protein results in more weight loss than from a diet with only 10 percent of the calories coming from protein. Therefore, based on this research, the following table lists the recommended amount of protein suggested per day, based on calorie requirements:

Daily Protein Needs Based on 15% of Caloric Requirements	
If your calorie requirements are:	Consume this amount of protein per day:
3000	112 grams
2800	105 grams
2500	94 grams
2200	83 grams
2000	75 grams
1800	68 grams
1600	60 grams
1500	56 grams
1200	45 grams

7) Eat Two to Three Meals Per Day With Minimal Snacking:

Why do we think that we need to eat three meals per day and snack between meals? This myth has led us to become fat and diabetic. The practice of eating six small meals became a practice when people with diabetes found their diabetes medications and insulin often caused blood sugar to drop too low. So they were encouraged to eat around the clock to avoid the lows. How crazy is that? Feed the lows, gain weight, increase insulin resistance from the weight gain, add another diabetes medication and another blood pressure medication, and then add a pain medication for the neuropathy that developed because of all the sugar that bathed the cells. That's the reality of this crazy practice of eating three meals per day and snacks between meals.

The goal is instead to limit the cells' exposure to carbohydrates and stop bathing the cells with sugar around the clock. Believe it or not, we really can get away with eating only two meals per day.

Many people do this all of the time on weekends. After a long five-day workweek, people often sleep in and eat a late breakfast. They don't eat again until dinnertime, and they are perfectly content. Why don't we do this during the week? Because our culture has trained us to eat three meals a day, we are exposed to food everywhere we go, and we are eating foods that increase our appetite and make us want to keep eating and eating.

Our ancestors were not surrounded by food everywhere they went. They would cycle through periods of feast and famine. Today we call this "intermittent fasting," and it has a positive impact on health and longevity. Intermittent fasting is not about binge eating followed by starvation or any other extreme form of dieting. Instead, intermittent fasting times meals to allow for regular periods of fasting. Intermittent fasting can be done daily, for a couple of days a week, or every other day. There are many variations of Intermittent fasting, but the one I like and personally use at least two times a week is to restrict eating to a specific window of time, in my case, an eight-hour window, so my fast is for sixteen hours. This might mean eating between the hours of 11 a.m. to 7 p.m. (preferably stopping at least two to three hours before bedtime). I have always practiced this style of eating on weekends, but I didn't know I was doing a fast. It's just how we eat on weekends. This might explain my really good metabolism all my life. There is no restriction of calories; just continue to eat the healthy way described in this book.

<u>Benefits of Intermittent Fasting</u>:

* Increases insulin and leptin sensitivity and boosts mitochondrial energy efficiency, while reducing the risk of chronic diseases, from diabetes to heart disease and even cancer
* Increases ghrelin levels, known as the hunger hormone, to reduce overeating
* Increases the ability to become fat-adapted, which increases energy by burning stored fat

* Increases the production of brain-derived neurotrophic factor (BDNF), a hormone that promotes brain health and protects against Alzheimer's disease and Parkinson's disease.
* Promotes human growth hormone production, which burns fat and has been shown to slow the aging process
* Decreases triglyceride levels, thereby decreasing risk of cardiovascular disease and diabetes
* Decreases inflammation and free radical damage (oxidative stress)
* Decreases weight gain and metabolic disease risk
* Decreases risk of dementia by the ketones that are produced as a result of fat breakdown; ketones, not glucose, are the preferred fuel for the brain.

It's really not difficult to eat in this fashion (or fast for this long) once you have trained your body to use fat as fuel, instead of sugar. And if you are not hungry, not eating for several hours is no big deal.

Whether you choose to eat two meals per day with the intermittent fasting model or choose to eat three meals per day, there are options for you to consume the proper foods between those meals. I don't like to use the word "snack," so let's instead use the term "meal extender." The snacks most people think of are cookies, fruit, crackers, chips, candy, etc. These types of snacks are off limits. Instead, your meal extenders are things like green tea (decreases appetite so have a cup between meals), a hard-boiled egg, a handful of nuts or a tablespoon of almond butter with celery sticks, a small salad, an avocado with olive oil and apple cider vinegar with pumpkin seed sprinkles, raw vegetables or a healthy jerky. In other words, choose a high protein/high healthy fat, low carbohydrate option for your meal extender.

Eating more than three meals per day is unnecessary; it can lead to constantly elevated blood sugar and insulin levels. Eat every four to five hours and give your digestion system a break between meals. Plain and simple: snacking is a bad habit and can be disastrous for blood sugar and insulin control as well as for weight management. On a three-meal-a-day schedule, eat your meal, then don't eat until the next meal (4-5 hours later).

8) **Eat Breakfast**:

If you are eating two meals per day on an intermittent fasting day, you may not call your first meal of the day "breakfast," although you are still "breaking the fast." Perhaps you prefer to call it "brunch." Whether you eat your typical breakfast foods or choose to eat brunch, lunch, or dinner foods for your first meal of the day, it's important that it be substantial and with minimal carbohydrates.

It's even more important for your breakfast to be substantial when you are eating three meals a day, especially if you go to an office where your efforts could be sabotaged by well-meaning co-workers bringing in donuts or other damaging temptations. You need to arm yourself well to avoid these temptations, and it's not hard to do when you know what to do.

Skipping meals, especially breakfast, can lead to increased food consumption throughout the day, can aggravate food cravings, and has been shown to increase nighttime eating habits. Of course, this depends on the quality of the breakfast, because cereal, milk, and fruit for breakfast just won't cut it, as I've said.

To assure a quality breakfast, include *all* of the following:

* One to two servings of a vegetable. Sauté spinach or broccoli or asparagus in an omelet or with poached, scrambled, or fried egg or kale. Blend spinach or broccoli in a smoothie.
* 1 tablespoon each of chia seed and flaxseed (mixed in a smoothie, breakfast pudding, or yogurt or "just as is" gulped down with water
* One to two servings of a protein. Think: eggs, salmon, other meat, or organic whey or pea protein powder blended in a smoothie

* One to three servings of a healthy fat, such as avocado or avocado oil, organic bacon, butter (you can cook your meat in these fats), or a nut butter
* One serving of fruit (optional), like ¾ cup berries, one kiwi, ½ banana

Flax seeds and chia seeds are nutraceutical foods. (Nutraceuticals are products derived from healthy foods that pack an extra health punch as a bonus.) These seeds provide part of your daily fiber needs and expand in your stomach to help you feel full and satisfied longer, while also providing all the benefits of healthy omega-3 fats. Whey and pea proteins are also nutraceutical foods. Whey protein helps to promote weight loss by reducing that pesky "hunger" hormone, ghrelin. Whey also helps lower blood pressure and acts as a natural ACE inhibitor (a type of pharmaceutical blood pressure medication). Other types of protein powders, like soy, don't have these benefits. Use pea protein if you have a milk allergy or sensitivities to whey or if you are vegan.

9) **Drink Intelligently**:

Here's where so many people get into trouble. They are drinking their calories without realizing the damage they are doing, or they are drinking calorie-free beverages. Both are highly discouraged:

a) *Ditch the Diet Sodas*

Trying to save some calories by drinking a calorie-free beverage, such as diet soda? You actually are causing the opposite reaction. New studies are now providing evidence that people who drink diet soft drinks do not lose weight. In fact, they *gain* weight! Keep in mind that these studies are correlation studies, not cause-and-effect, and signify that something linked to the diet soda drinking is also linked to obesity. For example, often people trying to lose weight will make a choice to indulge in a piece of cake and justify it because their diet soda saved calories.

However, the relationship between diet soda and weight gain is still much more than this. When we offer the body the sweet (artificial) taste of diet drinks but give it no calories, this alerts the body to the possibility that it has just consumed a nutrient. It will, therefore, search for the calories promised but not delivered. So you eat a piece of cake. We can't fool the body. Other studies do suggest that diet sodas stimulate appetite. All these negative effects of diet sodas are in addition to the harmful effects of artificial sweeteners in general.

b) *Ditch the Regular Sodas*

Sodas constitute the leading sources of added sugar in the diet of all Americans. I could go on and on about the dangers of soda and how they contribute not just to obesity and diabetes, but other health conditions, including osteoporosis, liver disease, heart disease, tooth decay, gastrointestinal distress, kidney stones and chronic kidney disease, heartburn, and acid reflux. Drinking a single can a day of sugar-laden soda may result in more than a pound of weight gain a month. It has been reported that for every soft drink or sugar-sweetened beverage a child drinks every day, their obesity risk jumps 60 percent. What makes sodas even worse for our children is the use of high-fructose corn syrup in place of the sugar in sodas, which contributes to liver disease. Can you believe this is even allowed?

I have been an outspoken critic of sodas since my children were in grade school. Over twenty-three years ago, when my children were only about 11 and 6, I approached the school board about removing the soda machines in their school. I was looked at as some nerdy parent making a big deal over nothing. The school board's response was that the schools needed money and the soda companies were happy to pay the school to sell their products. Needless to say, I lost that battle with the school board. In my opinion, the school system is as guilty as the soda companies for their role in creating the "diabesity" epidemic.

c) *Ditch the Juice*

There is absolutely no reason to drink juice. It's as bad as soda. Just because it comes from a fruit does not mean it is healthy. In fact, most processed juices contain high-fructose corn syrup, which you know by now is extremely harmful. Children today are getting way too much juice, which not only contributes to tooth decay but also obesity and liver disease. If you have to have juice, fresh squeeze it yourself, and go easy on the amount. You are always better off consuming the fresh fruit instead of the juice for all of its other health benefits, including fiber, pectins, and other antioxidants that are only found close to the rind or on the skins of the fruit.

d) *Ditch the Alcohol*

Keep alcohol to a minimum or preferably avoid entirely, even wine and especially beer. There really are no redeeming qualities of any kind to alcohol, and it will almost always lead to you consume more calories than you normally would consume, not to mention the calories that are in the alcohol. Forget all that you have heard about the benefits of resveratrol in red wine. You can never get enough resveratrol from wine, even if you drink ten glasses, which obviously would not be appropriate. Alcohol will also compromise the liver detoxification pathways, allowing toxins to build up in your body. If you do drink alcohol, keep it to just one serving per day, and make sure you are doing everything else you can to optimize your detoxification and elimination pathways (see Chapter 1).

e) *Enjoy Fresh, Natural Pure Water*

Our cells require pure, natural water to function properly. Every cell in the body requires water to survive. Water is used to remove waste products and toxins from the body, regulate body temperature, lubricate tissues and joints, provide natural moisture to skin and other tissues, cushion joints and help strengthen muscles, aid in the softening of stool for elimination, and help assimilate the nutrients in the food we eat.

For too many people, water is the forgotten nutrient. Some people substitute all of their water with other beverages, many of which are dehydrating beverages, such as caffeine and alcohol, which further increases fluid requirements. This is a serious problem. It's also the forgotten nutrient because people forget to drink it until it's too late (they are already dehydrated). We take it for granted that all water is the same. It's not. The water we drink today may be contaminated due to many factors. Pure, clean water is vital to keep our body systems running effectively and should not be taken for granted.

When it comes to weight loss, water is an extremely important nutrient, not only because it has no calories, but because it provides energy and helps to suppress appetite. Insufficient water will greatly slow weight loss if not halt it completely. Drinking half a liter of water (seventeen ounces) can boost your metabolism by 30 percent for one to one and a half hours. Drinking water cold is best because the body must expend energy (calories) to heat the water to body temperature. The best time to drink water is before meals.

Certain populations will require additional water considerations than others. These include the elderly, children, pregnant and breast-feeding women, and athletes or those engaging in physical activity. To determine how much water you should consume each day, divide your weight (in pounds) in half for the number of ounces of water you should drink. Divide that number by eight for the number of cups of water you need each day.

If you wait until you are thirsty to begin drinking water, you are already dehydrated and will need a half to one quart of water to get back into balance. Therefore, it is important to drink before becoming thirsty! Caffeinated and sweetened drinks cause even greater dehydration. Water is the only beverage we need, and it works the best for health and longevity.

How Pure is Your Water?

You can see how important it is to drink pure water. It is becoming increasingly difficult to find pure water. Our water supply has become potentially toxic with a prevalence of dangerous chemicals. Chlorine and fluoride are often added to the water supply for what is thought to be beneficial reasons, but these chemicals have toxic consequences. A wide range of other toxic and organic chemicals, largely from agricultural and industrial waste, contaminate the water supply, including PCBs, pesticide residues, nitrates, and even heavy metals, like arsenic, cadmium, lead, and mercury.

Tap water contains chlorine, which increases free radical damage, contributes to many forms of cancer, and increases the risk of high blood pressure. Chlorine also causes magnesium deficiency, which then causes increased urinary excretion of calcium and phosphorus, leading to the increased risk of osteoporosis.

If it wasn't for the high risk of agricultural chemical contamination, rural well water might be an ideal option. It is rich in magnesium and calcium, and drinking it would be like taking a daily mineral supplement. But another, more viable option might be to install an under-the-sink water filtration system. These systems effectively remove chlorine, bacteria, pesticides, and other organic chemicals by using a solid carbon block filter. The magnesium and calcium and other dissolved minerals are maintained. A reverse osmosis (RO) filter is ideal to avoid pharmaceutical residues.

Drinking and cooking with purified water is becoming more important. This includes having purified water to soak beans and nuts, to cook grains, and to steam vegetables.

So, there you have it: the B for Belly of *PRESCRIPTION DETOX: How Our Allegiance to Big Pharma Makes Us Sicker and How You Can Heal Without Meds*. I hope you will spend some time in your kitchen with an attitude of discovery and creativity. I know that if you take this very worthy task to heart, you will discover new things about yourself and realize just how strong you really are. You will delight in how your blood glucose and A1c results are plummeting, your waistline is shrinking, your energy levels are rising, your self-esteem is growing, and your blood pressure is normalizing. You will be on your way to a healthier and wealthier life, one that does not include pharmaceutical medications. I am very excited for you taking this very important journey of self-discovery. I hope you will celebrate your success and shout it out to the world!

PART 3: C is for Cell

Every thirty-five days, your skin replaces itself, and your body makes new cells from the food you eat. What you eat literally becomes YOU. You have a choice in what you are made of.

The "C" of the ABCs of *PRESCRIPTION DETOX: How Our Allegiance and Addiction to Big Pharma Makes Us Sicker and How You Can Heal Without Meds* is "Cell." For the body to heal, we must fix the cell. Which cell? All 37.2 trillion of them (according to a research study in the *Annals of Human Biology Journal*). Everything we are is comprised of these living cells that are constantly in the process of dying and replacing themselves as long as all systems receive what they need. The hair and nails are constantly growing, and our skin turns over every day. The entire outer layer of skin is replaced in about four weeks, and within a year the entire bone structure is rebuilt. However, the quality of the new cell replacing the old cell is totally dependent on the cells' exposure to the quality of nourishment and its protection from less optimal substances, including toxins from food and the environment.

Conventional medicine can't nourish or fix the cell with "*Insert name of medication.*" Unhealthy cells are not the result of an "*Insert name of medication*" deficiency. You will never be able to get off of pharmaceutical medications without first repairing the cell and keeping it well nourished and protected from environmental threats. As discussed in Part 1, toxins are constantly abusing your cells every day. It's not enough just to avoid the toxin. We have to repair the damage that resulted from oxidative stress and inflammation as a result of the toxins' presence, or healing will never occur. Also, as discussed in Part 2, our cells may also be damaged as a result of inadequate nutrients and fuel to our belly (body). Prescribing a pharmaceutical medication will serve only as a Band-Aid to reduce the symptoms that result from the damaged cell. The illness continues to fester and worsen, sometimes to the death of cells, because the cause was never addressed.

To fix the cell, we need a transformation. The cost of treating chronic disease in this nation has escalated to unsustainable economic conditions. According to the Centers for Medicare & Medicaid Services, in 2008 the U.S. spent 16.2 percent ($2.3 trillion) of its gross domestic product (GDP) on health care. Other sources report that this exceeded the combined federal expenditures for national defense, homeland security, education, and entitlement programs. If we don't change how we deal with health care, it is estimated that by 2023 annual healthcare costs in the U.S. will rise to over $4 trillion, which is equivalent to the cost of four Iraq wars, essentially bankrupting the country. Pharmaceutical medications are not the answer to ending this nightmare. The only way to solve this costly riddle of chronic disease is to no longer focus on the suppression and management of symptoms with pharmaceutical medications, but to address the underlying cause of the chronic disease.

As demonstrated in Parts 1 and 2, chronic disease is a food- and environment-driven phenomenon. Chronic disease is also driven by lifestyle and influenced by genetics. We can't change genetics, but we do know that our genes are influenced by the food we eat, our environment, and our lifestyle. Today we have the ability to determine our genetic make-up and influence gene expression by transforming our diets, lifestyle, and environment to prevent the development of disease. This cannot be done with pharmaceutical medications that are toxic to our system, consequently harming our genetic makeup and further inhibiting healing. Instead, as I said in the introduction, healing and repair of the cells will occur through the principles of functional medicine and the teachings of Hippocrates.

Functional medicine directly addresses the underlying cause of disease using a systems-oriented approach on a personalized level. It's not a cookie-cutter approach as used in conventional medicine. For example, if you go to your medical doctor for a complaint of heartburn, there is almost a 100 percent guarantee that you will be prescribed a proton-pump inhibitor such as Prilosec (omeprazole), Prevacid (lansoprazole), or other equivalent pharmaceutical medication. But if you go to a functional medicine specialist who knows that the cause of your heartburn may be different from another person's cause of heartburn, they will dig much deeper into your complaints, because the treatment plan for you might be completely different from someone else, based on your personal circumstances.

To find out the most appropriate treatment, the functional medicine specialist delves deep into your history, maybe even as far back as birth or prenatally, or even digging into your mother's health before your conception. Sounds crazy? It shouldn't. It's possible that if your mother took antibiotics while pregnant with you, this would affect her gastrointestinal health, and yours, as well. If you were delivered by cesarean section and bottle-fed instead of breast fed, your gastrointestinal system would have developed with different microbiota than someone who was delivered vaginally and breast-fed. These circumstances can directly impact your gastrointestinal health. Years of toxin burden via environmental factors, including your antibiotic use, your diet, your work environment, may have a direct correlation to your present complaint of heartburn. But these same circumstances are not necessarily found in someone else also complaining of heartburn. Therefore, the treatment for the same complaint may be completely different. Digging deep is what functional medicine specialists do—after all, there are 37.2 trillion cells in our body, and it's important that the correct cell or cells are repaired.

There are seven core principles that guide functional medicine, according to The Institute for Functional Medicine, of which I am a certified practitioner member:

Seven Core Principles Guiding Functional Medicine:

1) The biochemical individuality of each human being is acknowledged, based on their genetic and environmental uniqueness.
2) A patient-centered approach to treatment is incorporated, instead of a disease-centered approach.
3) A dynamic balance is the ultimate goal sought among the internal and external factors in a person's body, mind, and spirit.
4) The web-like interconnections of a person's internal physiological factors are addressed.
5) Health as a positive vitality is emphasized, not merely the absence of disease, and identification of the factors that encourage this vitality are searched for.
6) The promotion of organ reserve as a means of enhancing the health span, not just the life span, is a paramount goal.
7) Functional medicine is based in science.

CHAPTER 7

Find Clinical Imbalances in the Cell

"It's the life in food that gives us life."
~ Dr. Elizabeth Lipski, Functional Clinical Nutritionist

In the functional medicine model, practitioners partner with their patients to find and treat the underlying cause of disease and to prevent disease. This model addresses the whole person, not just symptoms. I look at seven biological systems to find any "core clinical imbalances" present that might marry the mechanism of disease with the manifestations and diagnosis of disease.

I share these core clinical imbalances to give you some insight into what a functional medicine practitioner considers in working with patients. It's a little technical, but I believe it is important to introduce you to the processes going on in your body and how addressing any imbalances can repair the cell and restore your health.

Seven Core Clinical Imbalances

1) How is the patient **ASSIMILATING** (moving food, oxygen, chemicals, and other substances between the body and the outside world)?

   – How are they assimilating their nutrients? In other words, are there imbalances in digestion, absorption, microbiota/ gastrointestinal system and respiration processes? Potential imbalances can be caused by irritable bowel syndrome, bloating, small bowel bacterial overgrowth (SIBO), gastroesophageal reflux disease (GERD).

- How is the patient assimilating oxygen? Is the respiratory function operating optimally?
- What are they assimilating through the skin on a daily basis (toxic compounds absorbed from skin care products, etc.)?

2) Are there **DEFENSE and REPAIR** mechanism (immune and inflammatory) imbalances?

- Inflammation is a primary component of this imbalance, and key environmental factors, such as allergens, toxins, stress, trauma, infection, lowered oxygen, drugs, and alcohol, will be investigated. Potential problems in this imbalance include food allergies, gluten enteropathy, chronic sinusitis, asthma, rosacea, psoriasis, yeast infection, mold, edema.

3) Are there imbalances in **ENERGY** regulation?

- We look at the imbalances caused by oxidative stress and mitochondrial damage. (Mitochondria are the powerhouses of the cells. They give the body energy.) Does the person have inadequate levels of antioxidants? What conditions might lead to energy dysregulation or a decreased amount of ATP (adenosine triphosphate, which transports energy in the cells for metabolism) or inadequate nutrition? An energy regulation imbalance can cause migraines, chronic fatigue disorders, fibromyalgia, pain, brain dysfunction, cognitive decline, and dementia.

4) Can the patient **BIO-TRANSFORM and ELIMINATE** toxins? What is this patient's total toxic load? We look at the organs responsible for elimination and clearance, the patient's nutrition,

and their genetic predispositions (ability or lack of ability to transform compounds and hormones). Problems in this imbalance might be due to fibromyalgia, multiple chemical sensitivities, mercury toxicity, and mercury dental amalgams.

5) Is the patient able to effectively **TRANSPORT** nutrients, hormones, fluid and other molecules throughout the circulatory (cardiovascular) and lymphatic systems? Once absorbed, nutrients must be distributed to the tissues for metabolism to occur. Defects in transport proteins, called lipoproteins, or specific genetic uniqueness can result in altered transport and distribution effects that alter a person's physiological function.

6) Is there effective **COMMUNICATION** of endocrine (hormone) signals, neurotransmitters, and immune messengers both outside and inside the cell? Potential problems in this imbalance can include insulin resistance, polycystic ovarian disease, hypothyroidism, estrogen toxicity, painful menstrual cycles, premenstrual syndrome, fibroid or uterine imbalance, and depression with anxiety.

7) Does the patient have **STRUCTURAL INTEGRITY** (replication, repair, and maintenance) of their sub-cellular membranes to the musculoskeletal system and the whole body level? We look at the patient's body composition, the integrity of the gastrointestinal system, and all cellular structures that define the self. Potential problems in this area might be osteoarthritis, rheumatoid arthritis, and osteopenia/osteoporosis.

Imbalances in these seven areas are the precursors to the signs and symptoms by which we detect and label (or diagnose) disease. The most important thing we do in functional medicine is to restore balance in the patient's fundamental physiological process and their environment.

CHAPTER 8

Core Lab Tests to Guide Cell Repair

"Symptom suppression is not the same as health prevention. Sick care is not the same as healthcare. Treating disease is not the same as treating people."
~ Dr. Russell Jaffe, Physician & Scientist

In the functional medicine world, diseases do not exist. Instead, focus is placed on a new map of core clinical imbalances and their patterns and connections to find the causes that lead to the clinical imbalances, and focusing on learning how to restore balance within the cells.

In this model, it is possible to see that one disease or condition may have multiple causes or imbalances, just as one fundamental imbalance may be at the root of many seemingly disparate conditions. For example, "obesity" is one "condition" that has many "imbalances" (e.g. inflammation, hormonal imbalance, mood dysregulation, genetics/epigenetics and diet/exercise). Whereas "inflammation" is one "imbalance" that can be the cause of many "conditions" (heart disease, depression, arthritis, cancer, diabetes).

Your healthcare practitioner should make an assessment of the seven core imbalances, along with a very deep, methodical personal and medical history to determine the most appropriate functional medicine laboratory tests to perform. Laboratory assessment is crucial in helping to get to the cause of the core imbalances. The cells are too fragile to throw just anything at them, especially potentially toxic pharmaceutical medications. It's always important "to test and not guess." The results from this sophisticated testing can better guide your practitioner in treating you for an optimal outcome.

Here are the lab tests your practitioner may consider to evaluate each of the seven core imbalances and to determine the most effective treatment plan for your condition. I share these with you not to overwhelm you but to help you appreciate the complexity of your body and understand the opportunity to identify deficiencies. If you are ready to stop guessing which supplements your body needs (and stop spending money on what may be useless), the right tests and an insightful interpretation by a qualified practitioner are essential to healing without prescription meds.

Assimilation

1) Protein/Amino Acid Assessment: This test helps to identify any metabolic imbalances underlying many chronic disorders by evaluating dietary protein adequacy and assimilation. The results can accurately identify nutritional deficits, metabolic impairments, and amino acid transport disorders, and then guide the appropriate treatment. Amino acids are essential for life. They are involved in neurotransmitter function, pain control, pH regulation, detoxification, cholesterol metabolism, and control of inflammation. Amino acids comprise the building blocks of the body's structural tissues and hormones. These compounds utilize or derive from the essential amino acids provided by the diet. Determining the adequacy of amino acids, the proper balance between them, and the conversion capability are of paramount importance to get to the root of many chronic disorders and prevent illness.

2) Advanced Lipid Assessment: This panel looks at elements that drive stubborn weight loss and blood sugar imbalances. This panel goes beyond standard cholesterol testing to give you cardiometabolic

and diabetes risk factors and markers of inflammation, including omega-3 fatty acids and insulin status. Standard cholesterol testing can give a false positive result, meaning that testing appears normal, thereby leaving you at risk for heart attacks, stroke, and diabetes. If cholesterol is elevated, a standard cholesterol test can lead to the inappropriate and unnecessary prescribing of cholesterol medications, when the actual problem is not cholesterol but inflammation, which can be remedied easily without medications.

This type of testing identifies risk factors for heart disease and stroke beyond cholesterol. These risk factors can be identified only with advanced lipoprotein testing. Cholesterol is carried through the body in little balls called lipoproteins, and it is the lipoproteins, not the cholesterol inside them, that lead to clogging of the arteries. Small, dense low-density lipoproteins (LDL) lead to the build-up of plaque that becomes oxidized and easily penetrates the arterial endothelium of the vessel wall.

A full lipid assessment will also assess lipoprotein(a), also called lipoprotein "little a," Lp(a), which is a small, dense LDL, an extremely atherogenic (harmful) lipoprotein strongly linked to thrombosis (blood clots). You may have heard it referred to as the "widow-maker." Lp(a) is largely determined by your genes, and if elevated, a very urgent and focused therapeutic plan is indicated. It is correlated with oxidized LDL. You want your Lp(a) to be less than 30 mg/dl.

This test also measures remnant lipoproteins (RLP), which are highly atherogenic (causing atherosclerosis) and are believed to be the building block of plaque. RLP does not need to be oxidized like other LDL particles to become dangerous. A measurement of HDL2b is also assessed and correlated with heart health, as it is an indicator of how well excess lipids are being removed.

An advanced lipid assessment should also provide information on your levels of inflammation in the entire body through measuring homocysteine and C-reactive protein (CRP) levels.

CRP is an indicator of inflammation throughout the body, including the cardiovascular system. Even in small amounts, CRP is associated with an increased risk of heart disease. High levels of homocysteine are associated with red blood cell aggregation, and also associated with low levels of vitamins B6, B12, and folate, and an indicator of poor lifestyle and diet.

3) Micronutrient and Antioxidant Testing: Conventional medicine has generally ignored assessing the micronutrient status of patients. This is a problem (and why you are reading this book), because vitamin and mineral deficiencies may be responsible for many chronic health conditions. With our Westernized "Standard American Diet" and contaminated and nutritionally-depleted food supply, we are a malnourished nation. We can no longer ignore our nutritional state and how it affects our health.

Vitamins have diverse biochemical functions. Some, such as vitamin D, have hormone-like functions as regulators of mineral metabolism, or regulators of cell and tissue growth and differentiation (such as some forms of vitamin A). Others, such as vitamin E and vitamin C, function as antioxidants. The largest number of vitamins, the B complex vitamins, function as precursors for enzyme co-factors that help enzymes work as catalysts in metabolism. Minerals are essential nutrients that function as co-factors in most biochemical reactions. A deficiency in just a single mineral can cause disease and upset hormonal balance.

Many people work at improving their health yet still have deficiencies due to:

a) Biochemical individuality: we are all metabolically and biochemically unique. The specific micronutrient requirements for one person may be quite different than the requirements for another.

b) Absorption: even if one eats a balanced diet, if the nutrients are not absorbed properly due to other dysfunction, deficiencies will develop.

c) Chronic illness: health conditions such as arthritis, cancer, cardiovascular disease, diabetes, fatigue, and multiple sclerosis can be affected, directly or indirectly, by micronutrient deficiencies.

d) Aging: our micronutrient requirements at age thirty are quite different from our requirements at age forty, fifty, and beyond. Absorption difficulties, especially of vitamin B12, quite commonly occur as we age.

e) Lifestyle: excessive physical activity, prescription drugs, smoking, alcohol, and sedentary habits all impact micronutrient demands.

4) <u>MTHFR Genotyping</u>: MTHFR (methyletetrahydrofolate reductase) is an enzyme that converts folic acid into the usable form our bodies need. It is a key enzyme in an important detoxification reaction in the body—one that converts homocysteine (which is toxic), to methionine, (which is benign). If this enzyme is impaired, this detoxification reaction is impaired, leading to high homocysteine blood levels. Homocysteine is abrasive to blood vessels, essentially scratching them, leaving damage that may lead to heart attacks, stroke, dementia, and a host of other problems. Additionally, when the enzyme MTHFR is impaired, other methylation reactions are compromised. Some of these methylation reactions affect neurotransmitters, which is why impaired MTHFR activity is linked with depression. Inefficiency of the MTHFR enzyme is also linked to migraines, autism, fertility, cancer, and birth defects, all of which depend on proper methylation.

A specific gene controls how well this enzyme works. A simple blood test can tell you if you have variant (dysfunctional) copies of the MTHFR gene. Fifty-one percent of the population have a least one variant MTHFR gene. If the MTHFR enzyme is inefficient, you can compensate for your body's inability to methylate efficiently since this biological process is dependent on several B vitamins. You may simply need more B vitamins, such as vitamin B6, B12 (methylcobalamin) and the active form of folate (5-methyl tetrahydrofolate), than someone without a variant copy of this gene. Other methyl donors such as SAM-e and trimethylglycine may also provide benefits. A methyl donor is a substance that can transfer a methyl group to another substance.

If you have a defective copy of the MTHFR gene, it is important that you monitor your homocysteine level. Fortunately, lowering homocysteine can often be done with the nutrient supplements listed above.

Determining what copies of the MTHFR gene you have gives you the ability to compensate accordingly. The old paradigm that we are simply at the mercy of our genes is now challenged. Genetic testing empowers you to take control, launching you into a new age of truly individualized healthcare.

5) Stool Testing for Digestion and Absorption and Microbiota: This non-invasive stool test will provide clinical value managing gut health, as it will include analysis of digestion, absorption, bacterial balance, inflammation, yeast, and parasites.

The integrity of the gut and digestive tract is most often the first place to start in a functional medicine approach to healing the body. Did you know that the area of the small intestine of your gastrointestinal tract is the size of a badminton course? Even though that is a lot of surface area for the absorption of nutrients, it is not unusual for it to become damaged and sick by daily exposure to toxins in our environment or food, or even by medications (including the overuse of antibiotics). If this is the case, nutrients are poorly absorbed, inflammation and autoimmunity occur, and over time we get aches, pains, and illnesses in other parts of our body.

Did you also know that your gut is your second brain? (Or is it your first brain?) There is a direct connection between your gut and neurological symptoms. Assessment of gut health is hugely important in getting to the cause(s) of health concerns. Gastro-intestinal imbalance can lead to Crohn's disease, ulcerative colitis, irritable bowel syndrome, and even to conditions beyond the digestive tract, including diabetes, obesity, rheumatoid arthritis, hormonal imbalance, depression, and chronic fatigue syndrome. Could the bacteria in your gut (or is it your brain), called the gut microbiome, be the cause of your health condition?

Stool testing can identify imbalances in bacterial flora in the large intestine, assess for parasites, *H. pylori* (a common infection of those with ulcers) and candidiasis (yeast) overgrowth, as well as issues with digestion and malabsorption, bacterial balance, and inflammation.

Common symptoms of gastrointestinal imbalance can include excessive gas or bloating, indigestion, burning, nausea, distention, loose stools, urgency, constipation, blood in the stool, pain, or cramping. However, a person can have gastrointestinal dysfunction without any gastrointestinal symptoms. Those with mood disorders, autoimmunity, autism, cardiovascular disease, obesity, and diabetes should also be tested.

6) <u>Omega-3/Omega-6 Fatty Acid Assessment</u>: Omega-3 and omega-6 fatty acids are polyunsaturated long chain fatty acids (PUFA) required by the body for proper functioning, normal growth, and the formation of neural synapses and cellular membranes. The omega-3 fatty acids have anti-inflammatory, anti-thrombotic, and antioxidant effects and can help reduce triglyceride levels. The omega-6 fatty acids have pro-inflammatory and pro-thrombotic properties at high levels. Analysis of omega 3- and omega-6 fatty acids is useful in chronic pain/inflammatory conditions, depression, cardiovascular risk, weight issues and for dietary guidance.

7) <u>Methylmalonic Acid (MMA) test</u>: This test may be used to help diagnose an early or mild vitamin B12 deficiency. It may be ordered alone or with a homocysteine test (mentioned above in the Advanced Lipid Test under Assimilation), as a follow-up test result that is at the lower end of the normal range. MMA is produced in very small amounts by the body and required for metabolism and energy production. In one step of metabolism, vitamin B12 promotes the conversion of a form of MMA, called methylmalonyl CoA, to succinyl Coenzyme A. If there is not enough B12 available, then the MMA level begins to rise, resulting in an increase of MMA in the blood and urine. This test is also including in organic acid testing (see below).

8) <u>Organic Acid Testing</u>: This is a urine test that provides information on how well your metabolism is working. Organic acids are formed as natural by-products of cellular metabolism, digestion of food, and by the metabolism of the gut microbes, e.g. bacteria and yeast. These organic acids can reveal if there are insufficient cofactors (e.g. micronutrients, like vitamins and minerals), that are critical for enzyme activity for metabolic pathways to proceed, or indicate the presence of candidiasis (yeast).

Additionally, this test can reveal:

* how well you are burning fat
* how well you are burning carbs
* how well you are converting food into energy
* how well you are methylating
* how well your liver is able to detoxify
* the level of oxidative stress, and thus the overall health of your cells
* if you have ample neurotransmitters, which have an effect on your ability to sleep, or affect your mood and/or tendency towards addictions.

Overall, this test is suitable for almost anyone, especially someone needing to produce more energy (due to overall fatigue, improve athletic stamina, promote weight loss, resolve depression, mood disorders or digestive complaints.

Defense and Repair

1) C-Reactive Protein (CRP): This is an "all-cause morbidity" indicator, I addressed above in the Advanced Lipid testing, which often includes this biomarker.

2) Erythrocyte Sedimentation Rate (ESR): This is a non-specific test that helps detect inflammation associated with infections, cancers, and autoimmune conditions. This test is often used in conjunction with the CRP. ESR is used to diagnose certain specific inflammatory diseases, temporal arteritis, systemic vasculitis, and polymyalgia rheumatic. A significantly elevated ESR supports the diagnosis. The ESR is also used to monitor disease activity and response to therapy in these diseases.

3) Food Allergy/Sensitivity Testing: The incidence of food sensitivities has increased dramatically over the years. It is estimated that up to 20 percent of the population have adverse reactions to foods. Increased total antigenic load related to food and environmental sensitivities has been associated with a wide range of medical conditions affecting virtually every part of the body. Mood and behavior, including hyperactivity disorders in children, are profoundly influenced by food allergies. A food sensitivity test assesses for specific antibodies, mainly IgG. Other tests assess IgA, IgM, or IgG4 antibodies. Some labs also test for IgE, which is a true allergy, compared to the other immunoglobins (Ig), which are measuring for sensitivities (not allergies). Think of immunoglobulins as your soldiers protecting you from foreign

invaders and each type of immunoglobulin as a different branch of the armed forces, e.g. Army, Navy, Air Force, Coast Guard.... you get the picture. Each branch has the same goal—to stop the invader—while each have a different role to accomplish this goal. The presence of these antibodies (the soldiers) indicates the presence of an enemy (aka a certain food).

4) Celiac Panel: Celiac disease (CD) is often undiagnosed and is caused in genetically predisposed individuals by abnormal intestinal permeability and abnormal immune response to gluten, a protein complex found in wheat, barley, spelt, and rye. The inflammatory autoimmune response damages the lining of the small bowel and is associated with diarrhea, bloating, fatigue, nutritional deficiencies, and systemic autoimmune conditions. Gluten sensitivity can cause similar symptoms but without the same level of tissue damage. This profile can help differentiate between CD, gluten sensitivity, and wheat allergy by evaluating the serum titers of IgA and IgG for tissue transglutaminase, deamidated gliadin peptide, and gliadin. Wheat allergy is assessed by titers of IgE for wheat.

5) Nutrigenomic Testing: Genetic variants are more common that we realized. More than 75% of all patients have significant genetic variations (SNPs) in the most important nutritional metabolism pathways. To avoid wasting money on nutritional supplements without knowledge or scientific proof of nutritional need or benefit, a genetic profile is beneficial. Without genetic validation of enzyme function, many supplements are not effectively delivered at the cellular level.

6) Celiac Gene Testing: This DNA testing can be done via blood or a cheek swab to determine whether an individual carries the genes responsible for the development of celiac disease. These

genes are located on the HLA-class II complex and are called DQ2 and DQ8.

7) <u>Stool Testing for Digestion and Absorption and Microbiota</u>: See "Assimilation" above.

8) <u>Lyme and Co-infection Panel Assessment</u>: A variety of tests are available for Lyme disease assessment, however, test results are sometimes ambiguous and therefore diagnosis must be made based on history and symptoms, as well as test results. Borrelia is most often the underlying infectious agent in Lyme disease, but there are other infections that may co-exist with Borrelia. Lyme disease has extensive neurological manifestations, causing cognitive, psycho-emotional, and behavioral changes. It is postulated that 20 percent of autism cases may be associated with Lyme disease. Lyme disease also has been linked as a possible cause of fibromyalgia, chronic fatigue, and arthritis.

9) <u>Viral Panel Assessment</u>: A viral test is done to find infection-causing viruses, which grow only in living cells and cause disease by destroying or damaging the cells they infect. They can damage the body's immune system, changing the genetic material (DNA) of the cells that infect or causing inflammation that can damage an organ. Viral tests may be done for viruses, e.g. Epstein-Barr virus (EBV), cytomegalovirus (CMV), respiratory syncytial virus (RSV), rotavirus, hepatitis, genital warts, herpes simplex, chickenpox, human immunodeficiency virus (HIV), and BK virus.

<u>Energy</u>

1) <u>Methylmalonic acid (MMA) test</u>: See "Assimilation" above

2) <u>Organic Acids assessment</u>: See "Assimilation" above

3) <u>Lactate/Pyruvate Ratio</u> (L:P): this is a helpful tool (but not diagnostic) for the evaluation of possible mitochondrial metabolism disorder. The mitochondria are the "powerhouses" or "brains" of the cell, responsible for creating 90 percent of the energy needed to sustain life and support organ function. When mitochondria malfunction, organs start to fail. The organs that require the greatest amounts of energy are the most affected: the heart, brain, muscles, and lungs. Symptoms can include strokes, seizures, and developmental delays; inability to walk, talk, see, and digest food; and a host of other complications.

4) <u>DNA Oxidative Damage Assay</u>: Oxidative stress is adversely involved in many pathophysiological processes, aging, and cancer. Oxidation of DNA occurs readily at the guanosine bases, so measurement of 8-hydroxy-2'- Deoxyguanosine (8-OHdG) in urine provides a quantitative assessment of ongoing oxidative damage or stress in the body. When 8-OHdG levels are elevated, it's important to identify the sources of oxidative stress and assess the primary intracellular antioxidant glutathione. Taking steps to reduce oxidative stress is valuable in optimizing health and longevity. This non-invasive test requires a single first-morning void (FMV) urine collection.

<u>Bio-Transformation and Elimination</u>:

1) <u>Detoxification Panels</u>

   a) <u>Phthalates & Parabens Profile</u>: This can help identify everyday exposures to toxins from the use of items such as personal care products and plastic food containers.

   b) <u>Organophosphates Profile</u>: This measures six dialkyl phosphates from a simple urine sample and indicates exposure to organophosphate pesticides. These toxins may be an underlying cause of health issues, including neurodevelopment and immune system disorders, ADD/ADHD, impaired memory, mood disorders, and increased risk of Alzheimer's disease and cancer.

c) Bisphenol A Profile: This determines exposure to bisphenol A (BPA), triclosanand 4-nonylphenol, which are considered endocrine (hormone) disruptors and are found in many of the products we use every day. Exposure to endocrine disruptors may play a role in obesity, adult onset diabetes, hormonal and neurological development disorders, and thyroid dysfunction.

d) Chlorinated pesticides: These can cause a range of illnesses, from allergies and asthma to cardiovascular disease and cancer.

e) PCBs Profile: This measures eight common PCBs that are shown to cause health problems with neurobehavioral and immune system development. Such problems may include psychomotor and behavioral problems, allergies, obesity, fatigue, and even some cancers. PCBs are stored in fatty tissues and accumulate over a patient's lifetime. Volatile solvents may cause symptoms ranging from blood disorders to muscular weakness and atrophy. These toxins may also be the underlying cause of many illnesses such as diabetes, fibromyalgia, brain fog and mood disorders, to name a few.

f) Volatile Solvents Profile: This measures exposure to common volatile solvents in our working and living environments.

g) Urine Glyphosate: High correlations exist between glyphosate usage and numerous chronic illnesses, including autism, hypertension, stroke, diabetes, obesity, Alzheimer's, dementia, Parkinson's, multiple sclerosis, kidney disease, thyroid disease, and others.

2) Heavy Metal Testing: Assessed via hair analysis, blood, first-morning urine or 24-hour urine tests, this test evaluates conditions that can result from heavy metal exposure, including autoimmune diseases, endocrine imbalances, neuropathies, and a host of women's conditions, e.g. endometriosis to infertility.

3) <u>Red Blood Cell Glutathione</u>: Glutathione (GSH) is the most abundant and important intracellular antioxidant. GSH in erythrocytes (red blood cells) is an indicator of intracellular GSH status, the overall health of cells and of the ability to endure toxic challenges. Low levels of GSH have been reported in cardiovascular disease, cancer, AIDS, autism, alcoholism, and debilitating neurodegenerative diseases such as Alzheimer's and Parkinson's diseases. It has also been associated with chronic retention of many potential toxic elements, chemicals, and some drugs. Assessment and support of erythrocyte GSH can contribute to healthy aging and effective detoxification of toxic metals and chemicals. This test is useful for assessing oxidative stress and aides treatment in conditions e.g. Alzheimer's disease, autism, cancer, cardiovascular disease, Parkinson's disease, and general health and longevity.

4) <u>DNA Oxidative Damage Assay</u>: See "Energy" above.

5) <u>Drinking Water Analysis</u>: to assure safe drinking water, it can be analyzed for pH and many elements including aluminum, antimony, arsenic, barium, beryllium, cadmium, copper, fluoride, iron, lead, manganese, mercury, nickel, selenium, thallium, uranium, zinc. More recently, there is a water test now able to detect glyphosate, the harmful active ingredient found in the herbicide Roundup.

6) <u>Glutathione Genetic Testing</u>: Glutathione is a major detoxification enzyme, responsible for clearing environmental chemicals and metabolic by-products from the body. Accumulation of these chemicals and by-products can damage intracellular biochemical functions. Alterations in these systems can have a significant negative effect on the nervous system and immune systems function. Genetic polymorphisms can result in decreased quality of life and even decreased life span.

Transport:

1) <u>Glucose Tolerance with Advanced Insulin Assessment</u>: This testing includes a snapshot of blood sugar at the time the lab is drawn, but also includes a Hemoglobin A1c, which is a marker of long-term glycemic control (over three months) and is also considered a marker of accelerated aging. An ideal assessment also measures C-peptide, which is an indicator of insulin production and can distinguish between types 1 and 2 diabetes. Insulin should also be measured, because it will provide clues about a person's insulin sensitivity. It can predict pre-diabetes or diabetes, if insulin is excessive, or if a person is making too little insulin, as a result of nutrient deficiencies, for example. Adiponectin, a hormone that enzymatically controls metabolism, is also ideally measured, with high levels being beneficial and an indication of efficient cellular energy production.

   This advanced testing also measures leptin, which is released by fat cells and helps control body weight through its effect on the appetite centers in the brain. Increased caloric intake, as well as increased body fat, leads to high leptin levels, which correspondingly causes an increase in hunger. Decreased caloric intake and decreased body fat cause a decrease in leptin, and therefore a decrease in appetite. Because obese people have larger fat cells, they produce more leptin so leptin levels tend to run high. Normally, elevated leptin levels would tell the body to stop eating, but obese people continue to eat, despite having consumed sufficient calories. This is a paradox called "leptin resistance." Because leptin levels are chronically high in the obese, in time the brain becomes resistant to (starts to ignore) its effects. Without the effect of leptin, the appetite-controlling factor that tells the body that it is full and not hungry is absent.

2) <u>Advanced Lipid Panel Assessment</u>: See "Omega-3/6 and Advanced Lipid Assessment" under "Assimilation."

3) <u>Breath Hydrogen-SIBO Assessment</u>: This non-invasive test detects bacterial overgrowth in the small intestine, a common condition that often overlies chronic symptoms of maldigestion and mal-absorption, including bloating, gas, diarrhea, irregularity, and abdominal pain. Normally, bacterial concentrations in the small intestine are minimal, but if they are excessive, the delicate mucosal lining is disrupted, including the microvilli that are responsible for nutrient absorption. Thus, serious health conditions can occur, including anemia, fibromyalgia, chronic fatigue syndrome, osteo-porosis, altered intestinal permeability (leaky gut), carbohydrate intolerance, malnutrition, and weight loss. Bacterial overgrowth can manifest silently, without overt clinical signs, and thus testing may be indicated, especially if the person has a history of constipa-tion, the use of acid-blocking medications, or maldigestion.

4) <u>Apo B/Apo A1-Particle Size Assessment</u>: Apo B (Apolipoprotein B100) is a measure of all atherogenic (harmful) lipoprotein par-ticles in the blood. ApoB is the protein core of LDL/VLDL (considered to be bad). ApoA1 is the protein core of the HDL (considered to be good). The desired goal for the ApoA1: ApoB ratio is to be less than 0.8. Higher can lead to an increased risk for cardiovascular issues.

Communication

1) <u>Thyroid Panel and Thyroid Antibody Assessment</u>: This blood panel determines thyroid function and can give more infor-mation to the diagnosis of hypothyroidism or hyperthyroidism. Fatigue, weight gain, sleep irregularities, hair loss, and disruption in skin health can all be signs of thyroid dysfunction. Also, this test includes key indicators to give a clear picture of thyroid function related to the inflammatory and autoimmune response of the thyroid gland.

2) <u>Saliva Adrenal Testing</u>: The adrenal glands, otherwise known as the "stress glands," enable our bodies to cope with stress and survive. Whether stress comes from outside in the form of a natural disaster or from within like the anxiety we experience before public speaking, it's the adrenals' job to help us adapt to the situation. They accomplish this by secreting key hormones: Cortisol, DHEA, and epinephrine/norepinephrine. Adrenals in balance produce adequate amounts of hormones to power us through the day. These hormones impact every process in the body, from energy production and immune activity to cellular maintenance and repair. They are key regulators of glucose, insulin, and inflammation and play a major role in bone and muscle building, mood and mental focus, stamina, sex drive, and sleep cycles.

Adrenals that are out of balance can lead to 1) high cortisol levels that result in insomnia, anxiety, sugar cravings, feeling tired but wired, increased belly fat, and bone loss; 2) low cortisol levels that cause chronic fatigue, low energy, food and sugar cravings, poor exercise tolerance or recovery, and low immune reserves; 3) out-of-balance DHEA (low or high), from which all sex hormones are derived.

3) <u>Neurotransmitters</u>: These brain chemicals facilitate the transmission of signals from one neuron to the next across a synapse and work with receptors in the brain to influence and regulate a wide range of processes such as mental performance, emotions, pain response, and energy levels. Functioning primarily in the central nervous system (CNS), neurotransmitters are the brain's chemical messengers, facilitating communication among the body's glands, organs, and muscles. Imbalances in certain neurotransmitters are associated with anxiety, depression, chronic fatigue, impulsivity, insomnia, and premenstrual syndrome.

4) <u>Gonadal Hormone Assessment</u>: These include the commonly known sex hormones that impact our mood, metabolism, and

cancer risk, including testosterone, estrogen, and progesterone. These also include important precursor hormones to testosterone and estrogens, such as DHEA-S, considered by many as the "mother hormone" since all other sex hormones are derived from it. The regulatory (peptide) hormones that control the production and release of other hormones are also tested here, e.g. follicle stimulation hormone (FSH) and luteinizing hormone (LH), which regulate reproductive health in both men and women. Sex hormone binding globulin (SHBG) and prolactin also are measured, both which may inhibit the action of major sex hormones like testosterone.

Regardless of gender, any of the following symptoms warrant an investigation to see if the gonadal hormones need optimizing—and optimization begins with nutrition or supplementation, not necessarily hormonal replacement: weight gain, insomnia, fatigue, hot flashes/night sweats, dry skin and hair, low libido, depression, anxiety, or diminished cognition, premenstrual syndrome, migraines or other pain, infections or autoimmune conditions, blood sugar dysregulation.

5) <u>Diamine Oxidase /(DAO)-Histamine Assessment</u>: DAO is the body's primary enzyme for breaking down ingested histamine and a natural defense against histamine excess. If you ingest too much dietary histamine or produce more than your DAO level can handle, reactions can occur. DAO is produced in the small intestine but certain drugs, foods, and bacteria may suppress its production. Low DAO levels are associated with migraines, chronic fatigue, hives, skin rash, eczema, psoriasis, nasal congestion, asthma, gastrointestinal disorders, inflammation, irritable bowel syndrome, premenstrual syndrome, estrogen dominance, arrhythmia, hypertension, hypotension, fibromyalgia, muscular pain, rheumatoid arthritis, neurological conditions (e.g. multiple sclerosis and attention deficit and hyperactivity disorder), depression, and anxiety.

Symptoms of low DAO are similar to those of histamine excess since it is the DAO that breaks down and metabolizes the histamine. People with the inability to break down histamine react to many substances and will often improve on antihistamines. Since DAO is made in the gastrointestinal tract, low levels are also indicative of poor digestive function and a compromised intestinal barrier.

Histamine is involved in many types of allergic and inflammatory processes, including immediate and delayed hypersensitivity reactions. It also acts as a neurotransmitter and regulates physiological function in the gastrointestinal tract. Histamine imbalances in the body may cause a variety of adverse effects ranging from life-threatening allergic reactions to localized itching, runny nose or hives. An excess of histamine may be a result of ingested histamine (certain foods), released histamine from storage sites in the body (from food or environmental triggers), or a diamine oxidase deficiency (needed for the breakdown of histamine).

Testing histamine along with diamine oxidase (DAO) levels provides important information that standard food sensitivity tests may not reveal. Often if food sensitivities are suspected, the culprit may be histamine intolerance. High histamine levels are associated with severe allergic reactions, low muscle tone, high blood pressure, dizziness, headache, nausea, vomiting, diarrhea, gas, intestinal cramps, painful menstruation, shortness of breath, congestion, runny nose, sneezing, hives, itching, flushing, abnormal heart rate. Low histamine levels are associated with: fatigue, depression, convulsions, seizures, sleep-wake disorders.

6) Insulin/Leptin Assessment: See "Glucose Tolerance with Advanced Insulin Assessment" under "Transport."

Structural Integrity:

1) Intestinal Permeability Assessment: This is a powerful noninvasive gastrointestinal test assessment of small intestinal absorption and barrier function in the bowel. The small intestine uniquely functions as a digestive/absorptive organ for nutrients as well as a powerful immune and mechanical barrier against excessive absorption of bacteria, food antigens, and other macromolecules. Both malabsorption and increased intestinal permeability ("leaky gut") are associated with chronic gastrointestinal imbalances as well as many systemic disorders.

   Increased intestinal permeability (leaky gut) of the small intestine can increase the number of foreign compounds entering the bloodstream and allow bacterial antigens (material foreign to the body like viruses, bacteria, food) to enter the bloodstream and cross-react with host tissue, thereby leading to an auto-immune condition. It can also enhance the uptake of toxic compounds that can overwhelm the body's detoxification system and lead to an overly sensitized immune system. On the other hand, decreased intestinal permeability is a fundamental cause of malabsorption, malnutrition, and failure to thrive.

   The Intestinal Permeability Assessment directly measures the ability of two non-metabolized sugar molecules to permeate the intestinal mucosa. The patient drinks a premeasured amount of lactulose and mannitol. The degree of intestinal permeability or malabsorption is reflected in the levels of the two sugars recovered in a urine sample collected over the next six hours.

2) Intestinal Antigenic Permeability Screen: This new technology for assessing leaky gut directly measures the integrity of the gut. It tests antibodies to markers and proteins involved in the intestinal barrier system. Thus, when there are elevated antibodies to one of these markers, there is a direct evaluation of compromise

to the intestinal barrier. This test also measures antibodies to lipopolysaccharides (LPS), which is the component of the membrane of gram-negative bacteria, which is a key underlying cause of leaky gut.

3) <u>Zonulin assessment</u>: Zonulin is a protein modulator of intestinal tight junctions used to assess intestinal permeability. Intestinal permeability plays a role in many chronic gastrointestinal and systemic conditions. Those who might benefit from a zonulin assessment are those experiencing gastrointestinal symptoms like bloating, gas, cramps, food sensitivities, joint pains, skin rashes and autoimmune conditions, or have gluten sensitivity, Celiac disease, or irritable bowel syndrome. Those with cardiometabolic diseases like types 1 and 2 diabetes, obesity, non-alcoholic fatty liver, and those with insulin resistance will also benefit from this testing.

4) <u>Red Blood Cell Fatty Acids</u>: The typical Western diet contains too many carbohydrates and saturated fats and is often imbalanced with respect to essential and nonessential fatty acid intake. Red blood cell fatty acid analysis is used to assess levels of and balance among the essential and non-essential fatty acids required for optimal health and wellness. Essential fatty acids regulate cell membrane integrity, blood pressure and coagulation, lipid levels, immune response, tumor growth and inhibition, and the inflammatory response to injury and infection. Red blood cell fatty acid analysis aids in developing the most effective dietary and supplemental treatment program to restore appropriate ratios among fatty acids.

5) <u>Quantitative Electroencephalography</u> (qEEG): This is the analysis of the digitized EEG (also called brain mapping) that measures electrical patterns (brainwaves) at the surface of the scalp. It is used as a clinical tool to evaluate brain function and to track

the changes in brain function due to various interventions, e.g. neurofeedback or medication.

6) <u>Event Related Potentials</u> (ERP): This is a non-invasive method of measuring brain activity during cognitive processing (e.g. the presentation of a word, sound or image). It is used to distinguish and identify psychological and neural sub-processes involved in complex cognitive, motor, or perceptual tasks.

7) <u>Brain Imaging</u> (also called neuroimaging): This uses various techniques to directly or indirectly image the structure, function, or pharmacology of the nervous system.

CHAPTER 9

Fix the Cell to Get Well

Wellness is not a 'medical fix' but a way of living - a lifestyle sensitive and responsive to all the dimensions of body, mind, and spirit, an approach to life we each design to achieve our highest potential for well being now and forever.
~Greg Anderson, Author & Cancer Survivor

In functional medicine, we do so much more than treat symptoms (and dispense pharmaceutical medications). We determine the cause of those symptoms and find the means to make the person thrive. In other words, with all of the data that is collectively gathered from a complete functional medicine assessment discussed thus far, two very important questions can be answered that will be used to guide treatment—fixing the cell.

1) <u>What does this person need to be rid of (or eliminated) or what is the primary cause of their symptoms?</u> These may include:

   a) Toxins: biologic, elemental, synthetic
   b) Allergens: food, mold, dust, animal products, pollens, chemicals
   c) Microbes: bacteria, ticks, yeast, parasites, infectious agents called prions
   d) Stress: physical, psychological
   e) Poor diet: the unhealthy food common to the "Standard American Diet"

2) <u>Does this person have unmet individual needs required for optimal functions?</u> What do they need to thrive?

   a) Foods: protein, fats, carbohydrates, fiber
   b) Vitamins, minerals, accessory or conditionally essential nutrients, hormones
   c) Light, water, air
   d) Movement
   e) Rhythm
   f) Love, community, connection
   g) Meaning or purpose

The primary purpose of therapeutic interventions is to prolong life, preserve functionality, and maintain maximum flexibility in the body. The approach to achieving these important goals is to normalize as many systems as possible using lifestyle, dietary change, supplements, hormones, and other holistic modalities, as appropriate.

Restoring balance in your environment and in the body's fundamental physiological processes is the key to cell repair and to restoring health and remaining free of the need for pharmaceutical medications. The treatment will be different for each person, regardless of the situation. Say goodbye to dispensing a pharmaceutical medication just because you have been told you have a specific diagnosis. To prevent or reverse disease will require the transformation of your diet, lifestyle, and environment.

The following are just a sampling of the tools that can be used to restore balance and repair the cell:

Lifestyle

<u>Diet and Nutrition</u>: It's no accident this is listed first. Remember, "food is medicine and medicine is food." Part 2 has covered this modality at length for the majority of people, but not all diets and

nutritional recommendations (including the ones in this book) are right for all people. Other considerations of the appropriate nutrition and diet for an individual will be based on their symptoms, genetics, and laboratory results. Specific therapeutic nutritional interventions may be needed, in addition to nutritional supplementation in the form of additional vitamins, minerals, and antioxidants.

Exercise: Not exercising or moving is a ticket to a slow death and ineffective healing overall. For those with limited movement ability due to back pain, breathing issues, musculoskeletal limitations, etc., it is crucial to seek a qualified practitioner for guidance in achieving regular and consistent movement.

Mind-Body

Self-Hypnosis: Hypnosis can allow the enhancement of communication and sharing of information between and within the mind-body. The body "hears" everything that enters the subconscious mind; thus your thoughts can be healing or destructive.

Relaxation Techniques: These are tools that can help balance the effects of stress while you work to reduce the problems causing the stress.

Heart Rate Variability Enhancement: The human heart does not beat at a steady rate, but rather fluctuates from beat to beat, which is called heart rate variability (HRV). In general, a high HRV is an indicator of health, whereas too little variability is a predictor of disease. Improvement in mental and emotional well being, including the ability to focus, improvement in listening ability, improvement in sleep, and a reduction in anxiety, fatigue, and depression have all been observed through the effective use of tools for improving HRV. These tools can be made available through your healthcare provider, or new "Bluetooth" technology can be delivered to your Android or iPhone that senses your overwhelm, anxiousness or scatteredness and allows you to shift and replace emotional stress with emotional balance and coherence. Go to http://heartmath.com for more information about this revolutionary technology.

Guided Imagery: These techniques teach psychophysiological relaxation to relieve pain and other symptoms, to stimulate healing responses in the body, and to help people tolerate procedures and treatments more easily.

Meditation: Meditation means being present with unmanipulated experience as it arises moment by moment. The practice of meditation serves your threefold physical, mental and spiritual health. It directly influences your ability to meet the challenges resulting from stress, burnout, and illness.

Biochemical

Probiotics and Botanical Supplements: Often these are required to repair the cell. Various health conditions have clearly benefited by specific supplementation of probiotics and botanical herbs. Both should be used on recommendation and monitoring of a functional medicine specialist, as they can have interactions and side effects with other medications or chemicals.

Detoxification: The importance of natural detoxification of the body was discussed in Part I, but often, based on symptoms and laboratory results, an intense detoxification plan may be indicated. This may or may not include chelation therapy, which should only be performed by a qualified practitioner. Chelation therapy is a process in which a synthetic solution is injected into the bloodstream to remove heavy metals and minerals from the body.

Essential Oils: These have been used for centuries for their aromatic properties and health-promoting benefits. Essential oils can support the body in many ways to promote optimal healing. Essential oils can promote healthy digestion, assist in healthy sleep patterns, improve cognitive function, and support immune function.

Hormones: It is the goal of functional medicine to return hormone levels to "normal" physiological levels in the most physiological way, preferably with bioidentical hormones if a hormone replacement is required. However, before replacing hormones, it is first necessary to correct the nutritional and environmental causes that led to the suboptimal hormone levels.

Biomechanical

Counterstrain: This is a technique used in osteopathic medicine, osteopathy, physical therapy, and chiropractic to treat muscle and joint pain dysfunction. The clinician uses only their hands to diagnose and treat tender points that are produced by inaccurate neuromuscular reflexes.

Acupuncture: This is the technique of piercing the skin with needles at specific points on the body to treat or prevent various conditions, including headaches, nausea and vomiting, musculo-skeletal conditions (of the bones and muscles), neck pain or other chronic pain, to improve sleep, relieve anxiety, and depression. Other conditions that benefit from acupuncture include allergies, asthma, sinusitis, sciatica, high blood pressure, sexual dysfunction, post-operative recovery, palliative care, chronic fatigue, menstrual irregularities, and even infertility.

Chiropractic: The nervous system dominates every cell of the body. Improper function of the spine due to slight misalignments (called subluxations) can cause poor healing or function, even in areas that are far removed from the spine and spinal cord. Misalignments can also reduce the ability of the body to adapt to an ever-changing environment. Even the slightest malfunction of the spine may alter the regular transmission of nerve impulses, preventing that portion of the body from responding optimally. Chiropractic uses spinal adjustments to correct misalignments and restore proper function to the nervous system, helping the body to heal naturally.

Give the body what it needs, and it will fix itself!

AFTERWORD

A lot of ground has been covered in these pages, but I have only scratched the surface. I have tried to simplify, as much as possible, how getting off meds and preventing chronic disease can be as easy as understanding your ABCs. Of course, I do understand that it is not as easy as we would like it to be. Living in our society today is difficult and stressful enough without worrying about all the toxins in our food and environment and how to feed ourselves for long-lasting health.

Just remember this: Do your best, because your best is always good enough! Keep working to get better and better. The human body is an amazing machine. If you give it what it needs and avoid what it doesn't, it will allow you to live a rich, productive, and fulfilled life and take you far on your journey to achieving all of your life's goals.

When the going gets tough, REMEMBER:

"No one ever complained about being too healthy!"
~ Cheryl Winter, Integrative Nurse Practitioner & Nutritionist

Thank you for allowing me to help you along your journey to greatness.

APPENDICES

APPENDIX 1

Clean Resources

Clean Food Resources

Environmental Working Group
Dirty Dozen: EWG.org/foodnews/dirty_dozen_list.php
Clean Fifteen: EWG.org/foodnews/clean_fifteen_list.php
Free Wallet Cut-Out Card: DiabeteStepsRX.com/wp-content/
uploads/2017/02/1_CFK_EWG_2016PesticidesInProduceGuide.pdf

For local farmers markets in your area, go to:
LocalHarvest.org
FarmMatch.com

Natural Resources Defense Council
Information on mercury in fish
NRDC.org/sites/default/files/walletcard.pdf

Non-GMO Shopping Guide
NonGMOShoppingGuide.com

Thrive Market
Online store for healthy snacks and personal care products
ThriveMarket.com

U.S. Wellness Meats
Quality grass-fed meat products (beef, pork, chicken, buffalo, and more)
GrasslandBeef.com

Vital Choice Wild Seafood & Organics
Safe seafood
VitalChoice.com

Matcha Source
Matcha green tea
MatchaSource.com

Nora's Food Company
Gluten-Free Granola & Snacks
NoraFoodCo.com

Against the Grain Gourmet
Gluten-free cookies, pizza, rolls, and baguettes
AgainstTheGrainGourmet.com

Hail Merry
Grain-free, vegan, non-GMO treats and desserts
HailMerry.com

Pete's Paleo
Grain-free meals delivered to your door
PetesPaleo.com

Cappello's Gluten Free
Grain-free pasta, cookie dough, and pizza kits
CappellosGlutenFree.com

Nick's Sticks
Grass-fed beef and free-range turkey jerky sticks
Nicks-Sticks.com

Steve's PaleoGoods
Grain-free snacks, bars, granola, and jerky
https://www.stevespaleogoods.com

Clean Cosmetics and Skin Care Resources

Annmarie
Organic skin care
AnnmarieGianni.com

W3LL People Cosmetics
W3llPeople.com

Red Apple Lipstick
Gluten-free, paraben-free lipstick and other cosmetics
RedAppleLipstick.com

Environmental Work Group
cosmetics products and ingredients database
EWG.org/skindeep

Native Deodorant
Aluminum-free and paraben-free deodorant
NativeCos.com

Air Purification Resources

IQAir
Whole-house air purifiers
http://iqair.com

Clean Home Cleaning Resources

Seventh Generation
SeventhGeneration.com

Real Simple
RealSimple.com

Greenshield Organic
GreenShieldOrganic.comEcover
Ecover.com

Grab Green Home
GrabgGreenHome.com

Mrs. Meyers
MrsMeyers.com

ECOS
Ecos.com

20 Mule Team
20MuleTeamLaundry.com

Dr. Bronner's Pure-Castile
DrBronner.com

APPENDIX 2

Guide to Eating Whole Foods

Eat whole foods. Avoid foods that are modern, processed, and refined. Eat as close to nature as possible, and avoid foods that cause stress for the body (blood sugar, digestion, etc.). Eat nutrient-dense foods to maintain energy levels. Enjoy your food, and eat in a relaxing atmosphere.

MEAT, SEAFOOD & EGGS

Including but not limited to:

- Beef
- Bison
- Boar
- Buffalo
- Chicken
- Duck
- Eggs
- Game meats
- Goat
- Goose
- Lamb
- Mutton
- Ostrich
- Pork
- Quail

- Rabbit
- Squab
- Turkey
- Veal

SEAFOOD:

- Catfish
- Carp
- Clams
- Grouper
- Halibut
- Herring
- Lobster
- Mackerel
- Mahi

- Mussels
- Oysters
- Salmon
- Sardines
- Scallops
- Prawns
- Snails
- Snapper
- Swordfish
- Trout

FATS & OILS

- Avocado oil
- Bacon fat/lard
- Butter
- Coconut milk
- Coconut Oil
- Duck fat
- Ghee
- Macadamia oil
- Olive oil: cold-pressed

- Palm Oil
- Schmaltz
- Sesame oil: cold-pressed
- Suet
- Tallow
- Walnut oil

VEGETABLES

- Artichokes
- Asparagus
- Arugula
- Bamboo shoots
- Beets
- Bok choy
- Broccoli
- Brussels sprouts
- Cabbage
- Carrots
- Cassava
- Cauliflower
- Celery*
- Chard
- Collard greens*
- Cucumbers
- Daikon
- Dandelion greens
- Eggplant
- Endive
- Fennel
- Garlic
- Green Beans
- Jicama
- Kale
- Kohlrabi
- Leeks
- Lettuce*
- Lotus roots
- Mushrooms
- Mustard greens
- Okra
- Onions
- Parsley
- Parsnips
- Peppers*
- Potatoes*
- Radicchio
- Radishes
- Rapini
- Rutabagas
- Seaweed
- Shallots
- Snap peas
- Spinach*
- Squash
- Sugar snaps
- Sunchokes
- Sweet potatoes
- Taro
- Tomatillo
- Tomatoes
- Turnip greens
- Turnips
- Watercress
- Yams
- Yuccas

* Buy Organic

FRUITS

- Apples*
- Apricots
- Avocados
- Bananas
- Blackberries
- Blueberries*
- Cherries*
- Cranberries
- Figs
- Grapefruit
- Grapes*
- Guavas
- Kiwis
- Lemons
- Limes
- Lynchees
- Mangoes
- Melons
- Nectarines*
- Oranges
- Papayas
- Passionfuit
- Peaches*
- Pears*
- Persimmons
- Pineapples
- Plantains
- Plums
- Pomegranates
- Raspberries
- Rhubard
- Star fruit
- Strawberries*
- Tangerines
- Watermelon

* **Buy Organic**

HERBS & SPICES

- Anise
- Annatto
- Basil
- Bay leaf
- Caraway
- Cardamom
- Carob
- Cayenne pepper
- Celery seed
- Chervil
- Chicory
- Chili pepper
- Chipotle powder
- Chives
- Cilantro
- Cinnamon
- Clove
- Coriander
- Cumin
- Curry
- Dill
- Fennel
- Fenugreek
- Galangal
- Garlic
- Ginger
- Horseradish
- Juniper berry
- Kaffir lime leaves
- Lavender
- Lemongrass
- Lemon verbena
- Licorice
- Mace
- Marjoram
- Mint
- Mustard
- Oregano
- Paprika
- Parsley
- Pepper, black
- Peppermint
- Rosemary
- Saffron
- Spearmint
- Star anise
- Tarr
- Thyme
- Tumeric
- Vanilla
- Wasabi
- Za'atar

NUTS & SEEDS
- Almonds
- Brazil nuts
- Chestnuts
- Hazelnuts
- Macadamia
- Pecans
- Pinenuts
- Pistachios
- Pumpkin seeds
- Sesame seeds
- Sunflower seeds
- Walnuts

LIQUIDS
- Almond milk, fresh
- Coconut milk
- Coconut water
- Herbal tea
- Mineral water
- Water

GRASS-FED DAIRY:
- Butter
- Ghee

BONE BROTH:
- Homemade only

ORGAN MEATS:
- Liver, kidneys, heart, etc.

SEA VEGETABLES:
- Dulse, kelp, seaweed

FERMENTED FOODS:
- Sauerkraut, carrots, beets, high-quality yogurt, kefir, kombucha

Source: Diane Sanfilippo (BalancedBites.com)

APPENDIX 3

Guide to Food Quality

Seek out REAL, whole food as much as possible. This includes foods without health claims on the packages. Better yet, DITCH the packaged food all together. Think produce and butcher counter meats and seafood.

MEAT, EGGS & DAIRY

BEEF & LAMB
Best! 100% grass-fed and finished, pasture-raised, local
Better: grass-fed, pasture-raised
Good: organic
Baseline: commercial (hormone/antibiotic-free)

PORK
Best! pasture-raised, local
Better: free-range, organic
Good: organic
Baseline: commercial

EGGS & POULTRY
Best! pasture-raised, local
Better: free range, organic
Good: cage-free, organic
Baseline: commercial

DAIRY
ALWAYS BUY FULL-FAT
Best! grass-fed, raw/unpasteurized
Better: raw/unpasteurized
Good: grass-fed
Baseline: commercial or organic
—*not recommended*

WHAT THE LABELS ON MEAT, EGGS & DAIRY MEAN

PASTURE-RAISED

Animals can roam freely in their natural environment where they are able to eat nutritious grasses and other plants or bugs/grubs that are part of their natural diet. There is no specific pasture-raised certification, though certified organic meat must come from animals that have continuous access to pasture regardless of use.

CAGE-FREE

"Cage-Free" means uncaged inside barns or warehouses, but they generally do not have access to the outdoors. Beak cutting is permitted. There is no third party auditing.

ORGANIC

Animals may not receive hormones/antibiotics unless in the case of illness. They consume organic feed and have outdoor access but may not use it. Animals are not necessarily grass-fed. Certification is costly and some reputable farms are forced to forego it through third party auditing.

NATURAL

"Natural" means minimally processed, and companies use this word deceivingly. All cuts are, by definition, minimally processed and free of flavorings and chemicals.

FREE-RANGE/ROAMING

Poultry must have access to the outdoors at least 51% of the time, and ruminants may not be in feedlots. There are no restrictions regarding what the birds can be fed. Beak cutting and forced molting through starvation are permitted. There is no third party auditing.

NATURALLY RAISED

"Naturally Raised," is a USDA verified term. It generally means raised without growth-promoters or unnecessary antibiotics. It does not indicate welfare or diet.

NO ADDED HORMONES

It is illegal to use hormones in raising poultry or pork;

therefore, the use of this phrase on poultry or pork is a marketing ploy.

VEGETARIAN-FED

"Vegetarian Fed" implies that the animal feed is free of animal by-products but isn't federally inspected. Chickens are not vegetarians, so this label on chicken or eggs only serves to indicate that the chickens were not eating their natural diet.

FATS & OILS

SEE THE FATS & OILS GUIDE FOR DETAILS.

Best! organic, cold-pressed, and from well-raised animal sources
Better: organic, cold-pressed
Good: organic or conventional

SEAFOOD

Best! wild fish
Better: wild-caught
Good: humanely harvested, non-grain-fed
Baseline: farm raised—*not recommended*

WILD FISH/WILD-CAUGHT FISH

"Wild fish" indicated that the fish was spawned, lived in, and was caught in the wild. "Wild-caught fish" may have been spawned or lived some part of their lives in a fish farm before being returned to the wild and eventually caught. The Montery Bay Aquarium maintains a free list of the most sustainable seafood choices on their website.

NUTS & SEEDS

KEEP NUTS & SEEDS COLD FOR FRESHNESS

Best! local, organic, kept cold
Better: local, organic
Good: organic
Baseline: conventional

PRODUCE

Best! local, organic, and seasonal
Better: local and organic
Good: organic or local
Baseline: conventional

WHEN TO BUY ORGANIC:

Buy organic as often as possible, prioritize buying the Environmental Working Group's "The Dirty Dozen" as organic versus "The Clean Fifteen" -visit: www.ewg.org for details

PRODUCE SKUs:

Starts with 9 = organic - ideal
Starts with 3 or 4 = conventionally grown Starts with 8 = genetically modified
(GMO) or irradiated - avoid

Source: Diane Sanfilippo (BalancedBites.com)

APPENDIX 4

Low Carbohydrate Recipe Websites

DiabeteStepsRX.com/carbohydrate-controlled-recipes

BalancedBites.com/recipes

PaleoPlan.com

PaleoMom.com

Detoxinista.com

ElanasPantry.com

CupcakesOMG.blogspot.com/p/recipes.html

AgainstAllGrain.com/recipe-index

GlutenFreeAndMore.com

APPENDIX 5

Guide to Gluten

What is it? Gluten is a protein found in wheat, rye oats, and barley. Gluten is the composite of a prolamin and a glutelin, which exist, conjoined with starch, in the endosperm of various grass-related grains. Gliadin, water-soluble, and glutenin, water-insoluble, (the prolamin and glutelin from wheat) compose about 80% of the protein contained in wheat seed. Being insoluble in water, they can be purified by washing away the associated starch. Worldwide, gluten is a source of protein, both in foods prepared directly from sources containing it, and as an additive to foods otherwise low in protein.

SOURCES OF GLUTEN or items that may contain hidden gluten

- Ales
- Barley
- Barley malt/extract
- Beer & lagers
- Bran
- Breading
- Broth
- Brown rice syrup
- Bulgur
- Candy coating
- Communion "wafers"
- Couscous
- Croutons
- Durum
- Einkorn
- Emmer
- Farina
- Farro
- Gloss & balms
- Graham flour
- Herbal blends
- Imitation seafood
- Kamut
- Lipstick
- Luncheon meats
- Malt
- Makeup
- Marinades
- Matzo flour/meal
- Meat/sausages
- Medications
- Orzo
- Panko
- Pasta
- Play dough
- Roux
- Rye
- Sauces
- Seitan
- Self-basting poultry
- Semolina
- Soup base
- Soy sauce
- Spelt
- Spice blends
- Stuffing

- Supplements
- Thickeners
- Udon
- Vinegar (malt only)
- Vital wheat gluten
- Vitamins
- Wafers
- Wheat
- Wheat bran
- Wheat germ
- Wheat starch

GLUTEN-FREE*
(but still not recommended)

*Nearly all processed foods and grains carry some risk of cross-contamination. For the safest approach to a gluten-free diet, eat only whole, unprocessed foods.

- Amaranth
- Arrowroot
- Buckwheat
- Corn
- Flax
- Millet
- Montina™
- Nut flour
- Bean flour
- Potato flour
- Potato starch
- Quinoa
- Rice
- Rice bran
- Sago
- Seed flour
- Sorghum
- Soy (soya)
- Tapioca
- Teff

SIGNS OF GLUTEN EXPOSURE

- Abdominal bloating
- Fatigue
- Skin problems or rashes
- Diarrhea or constipation
- Irritable, moody
- Change in energy levels
- Unexpected weight loss, mouth ulcers, depression, and even Crohn's disease are all more severe gluten allergy symptoms that you may experience.
- Consult with your nutritionist or physician if you experience symptoms of a gluten exposure that result in prolonged discomfort.

MOST COMMON SOURCES OF HIDDEN GLUTEN

ALCOHOL:
Beer, malt beverages, grain alcohols

COSMETICS:
Check ingredients on makeup, shampoo, and other personal care items

DRESSINGS:
Thickened with flour or other additives

FRIED FOODS:
Cross contamination with breaded items in fryers

VINEGAR:
Malt varieties

MEDICATIONS, VITAMINS, AND SUPPLEMENTS:
Ask the pharmacist and read the labels closely

PROCESSED / PACKAGED FOODS:
Additives often contain gluten

SAUCES, SOUPS, AND STEWS:
Thickened with flour

SOY, TERIYAKI, AND HOISIN SAUCES:
Fermented with wheat

GLUTEN-FREE BOOZE**

- Brandy
- Bourbon
- Cognac
- Gin
- Grappa
- Rum
- Sake
- Scotch
- Sherry
- Tequila
- Vermouth
- Vodka
- Whiskey
- Wine
- Champagne
- Mead
- Hard cider
- Gluten-free beers

For travel gluten-guides, visit: www.celiactravel.com

FOR MORE INFORMATION ON GLUTEN

Additional resources to provide you ample information
if needing to be 100% strictly gluten-free.

- celiac.com
- celiac.org
- celiaccentral.org
- celiaclife.com
- celiactravel.com
- celiacsolution.com
- elanaspantry.com
- glutenfreegirl.com
- surefoodsliving.com

"**According to celiac.com, all distilled alcohols are gluten-free but
for someone with overt Celiac Disease, avoiding alcohols made from
wheat, barley, and rye is still recommended.

Source: Diane Sanfilippo (BalancedBites.com)

APPENDIX 6

Guide to Sweeteners

Ideally, sugar needs to be avoided and Artifical Sweeteners should never be consumed. For treats and special occasions, see the "natural Use Sparingly" selection. Sweeteners should not be considered "food" or nourishment.

NATURAL USE SPARINGLY

PREFERRED CHOICES ARE IN BOLD. USE ORGANIC FORMS WHENEVER POSSIBLE

- Brown sugar
- **Dates (whole)**
- Date sugar
- Date syrup
- Cane sugar
- Raw sugar
- Turbinado
- Cane juice
- Cane juice crystals
- Coconut nectar
- Coconut sugar/crystals
- **Fruit juice (real, fresh)**
- **Fruit juice concentrate**
- **Honey (raw)**
- **Maple syrup (grade b)**
- **Molasses**
- Palm sugar
- **Stevia (green leaf or extract)**

NATURAL BUT NOT RECOMMENDED

- Agave
- Agave nectar
- Barley malt
- Beet sugar
- Brown rice syrup
- Buttered syrup
- Caramel
- Carob syrup
- Corn syrup
- Corn syrup solids
- Demerara sugar
- Dextran
- Dextrose
- Diastatic malt
- Diastase
- Ethyl maltol
- Fructose
- Glucose / glucose solids
- Golden sugar
- Golden syrup
- Grape sugar
- High fructose corn syrup
- Invert sugar
- Lactose
- Levulose
- Light brown sugar

- Maltitol
- Malt syrup
- Maltodextrin
- Maltose
- Mannitol
- Muscovado
- Refiner's syrup
- Sorbitol

- Sorghum syrup
- Sucrose
- Treacle
- Yellow sugar
- Xylitol (or other sugar alcohols, typically they end in "-ose")

ARTIFICIAL
NEVER CONSUME

- Acesulfame K (Sweet One)
- Aspartame (Equal, Nutra-Sweet)
- Saccharin (Sweet'N Low)

- Stevia: white/ bleached (Truvia, Sun Crystals)
- Sucralose (Splenda)
- Tagatose

Source: Diane Sanfilippo (BalancedBites.com)

APPENDIX 7

Guide to Choosing Fats and Oils

Choosing the right fats & oils is essential for reducing inflammation & improving your health from the inside out. Limit eating out to assure you are avoiding harmful fats & oils. Avoid overly processed and refined forms of fats and oils & opt for organic whenever possible.

EAT THESE:
HEALTHY, NATURALLY OCCURRING,
MINIMALLY PROCESSED FATS

SATURATED: FOR HOT USES

BUY ORGANIC, UNREFINED FORMS
- Coconut oil
- Palm oil

IDEALLY FROM PASTURE-RAISED, GRASS-FED, ORGANIC SOURCES
- Butter
- Ghee, clarified butter
- Lard, bacon grease (pork fat)
- Tallow (beef fat)
- Duck fat
- Schmaltz (chicken fat)
- Lamb fat
- Full-fat dairy
- Eggs, meat, and seafood

Source: Diane Sanfilippo (BalancedBites.com)

UNSATURATED: FOR COLD USES

BUY ORGANIC, EXTRA-VIRGIN, AND COLD-PRESSED FORMS

- Olive oil
- Sesame oil
- Macadamia nut oil
- Walnut oil
- Avocado oil
- Nuts & seeds (including nut & seed butters)
- Flax seed oil**

NOTE: Unsaturated fats (typically liquid at 68 degrees room temperature) are easily damaged/oxidized when heat is applied to them. Do not consume damaged fats.

**Cold-pressed flax seed oil is okay for occasional use but supplementing with it or doses of 1-2 tablespoons per day is *not* recommended as overall PUFA

(polyunsaturated fatty acid) intake should remain minimal.

DITCH THESE:
UNHEALTHY, MAN-MADE FATS & REFINED SEED OILS ARE NOT RECOMMENDED

Hydrogenated or partially hydrogenated oils, as well as manmade trans-fats or "buttery spreads" like Earth Balance, Benecol, and I Can't Believe It's Not Butter are not healthy. These oils are highly processed and oxidize easily via one or more of the following: light, air, or heat.

- Margarine/buttery spreads
- Canola oil (also known as rapeseed oil)
- Corn oil
- Vegetable oil
- Soybean oil
- Grapeseed oil
- Sunflower oil
- Safflower oil
- Rice bran oil
- Shortening made from one or more of the above-listed "ditch" oils

APPENDIX 8

Guide to Cooking with Fats and Oils

Choose based on (in this order of importance):
1. How processed they are—the minimally processed the better—choose naturally occurring fats & oils
2. Their fatty acid composition—the more saturated they are, the more stable they are & the less likely to be damaged or oxidized
3. Smoke point—above this point the fats will become damaged & oxidized so stay below this temperature

ITEM NAME	%SFA	%MUFA	%PUFA	SMOKE POINT UNREFINED/ REFINED
Best Bets - Recommended for high-heat cooking THE MOST STABLE FATS				
Coconut oil	86	6	2	350/450
Butter/ghee	63	26	.03	300/480
Cocoa butter	60	35	5	370
Tallow/Suet (beef fat)	55	34	.03	400
Palm oil	54	42	.10	455
Lard/Bacon fat (pork fat)	39	45	11	375
Duck fat	37	50	13	375
Okay - For very low-heat cooking MODERATELY STABLE FATS				
Avocado oil*	20	70	10	520
Macadamia nut oil*	16	80	4	410
Olive oil*	14	73	11	375
Peanut oil**	17	46	32	320/450
Rice Bran oil**	25	38	37	415

Not recommended for cooking VERY UNSTABLE FATS			
Safflower oil**	8	76	13	225/510
Sesame seed oil*	14	40	46	450
Canola oil**	8	64	28	400
Sunflower oil**	10	45	40	225/440
Vegetable shortening**	34	11	52	330
Corn oil	15	30	55	445
Soybean oil	16	23	58	495
Walnut oil*	14	19	67	400
Grapeseed oil	12	17	71	420

SFA - saturated fatty acid
MUFA - monounsaturated fatty acid
PUFA - polyunsaturated fatty acid

* While not recommended for cooking, cold-pressed nut and seed oils that are stored in the refrigerator may be used to finish recipes or after cooking is completed—for flavor purposes.

** While the fatty acid profile of these oils may seem appropriate at first glance, the processing method by which they are made negates their healthfulness—they are not recommended for consumption, neither hot nor cold.

Source: Diane Sanfilippo (BalancedBites.com)

BIBLIOGRAPHY

Alazraki, M. (2010). Where do new drugs come from? U.S. biotech lead the way. Retrieved from https://www.aol.com/article/2010/11/30/where-do-new-drugs-come-from-u-s-biotechs-lead-the-way/19709158/

American Heart Association (2017). Heart disease and stroke statistics. Retrieved from https://www.heart.org/idc/groups/ahamah-public/@wcm/@sop/@smd/documents/downloadable/ucm_491265.pdf

American Diabetes Association (2017). *Statistics about diabetes.* http://diabetes.org/diabetes-basics/statistics/

Avena, N.M., Rada, P., and Hoebel, B.G. (2008). Evidence for sugar addiction: behavioral and neurochemical effects of intermittent, excessive sugar intake. *Neurosci Biobehav Rev, 32(*1), 20-39.

Ayas, N.T., et al. (2003). A prospective study of sleep duration and coronary heart disease in women. *Arch Intern Med, 163*(2), 205-9.

Bailey, H.D., et al. (2014). Parental occupational pesticide exposure and the risk of childhood leukemia in the offspring: findings from the childhood leukemia international consortium. *Int J Cancer, 135(*9), 2157-2172. doi: 10.1002/ijc.28854 Retrieved from https://www.ncbi.nlm.nih.gov/pmc/articles/PMC4845098/

Baltazar, M.T., et al. (2014). Pesticides exposure as etiological factors of Parkinson's disease and other neurogenerative diseases—A mechanistic approach. *Toxicology Letters, 230*(2), 85-103. doi.org/10.1016/j. toxlet.2014.01.039 Retrieved from http://www.sciencedirect.com/ science/article/pii/S0378427414000599

Bouchard, M.F., Bellinger, D.C., Wright, R.O., & Weisskopf, M.G.(2010). Attention-deficit/hyperactivity disorder and urinary metabolites of organophosphate pesticides. *Pediatrics, 125*(6). Retrieved from http://pediatrics.aappublications.org/content/ pediatrics/125/6/e1270.full.pdf

Budnitz, D.S., Pollock, D.A., Weidenbach, K.N., et al. (2006). National surveillance of energy department visits for outpatient adverse drug events. JAMA, 296(15), 1858-1866. doi:10.1001/ jama.296.15.1858 Retrieved from http://jamanetwork.com/journals/ jama/fullarticle/203690

Budnitz, D.S., Lovegrove, M.C., Shehab, N., and Richards, C.L. (2011). Emergency hospitalizations for adverse drug events in older Americans. N Engl J Med, 365, 2002-2012. doi: 10.1056/NEJMsa1103053 Retrieved from http://www.nejm.org/doi/full/10.1056/ NEJMsa1103053#t=article

Bray, G.A. and Popkin, B.M. (2014). Dietary sugar and body weight: have we reached a crisis in the epidemic of obesity and diabetes?: health be damned! Pour on the sugar. Diabetes Care, 37(4), 950-6. doi: 10.2337/dc13-2085

Brazanno, L.A., He, J., Ogden, L.G., Loria, C.M., Welton, P.K., and National Health and Nutrition Examination Survey (2003). Dietary fiber intake and reduced risk of coronary heart disease in U.S. men and women: the National Health and Nutrition Examination Survey, Epidemiologic Follow-up Study. *Arch Intern Med, 163*(16), 1897-904.

Centers for Disease Control and Prevention (2016). *Chronic disease overview.* https://www.cdc.gov/chronicdisease/overview/

Centers for Disease Control and Prevention (2017). Cancer statistics. Retrieved from https://www.cdc.gov/nchs/fastats/cancer.htm

Centers for Disease Control, National Center for Environmental Health (2012). *Second national report on biochemical indicators of diet and nutrition in the U.S. population.* Retrieved from https://www.cdc.gov/nutritionreport/pdf/nutrition_book_complete508_final.pdf

Cook, K. (2012). Autism Research Institute Conference. *10 Americans.* Retrieved from http://www.autism.com/index.php/webinars/cook_2012

Cyrex Laboratory (2017). *Specialty diagnostic laboratory testing.* https://cyrexlabs.com

Davidson, M.H., et al. (2011). Clinical utility of inflammatory markers and advanced lipoprotein testing: advice from an expert panel of lipid specalists. J Clin Lipidol, 5(5), 338-67. doi: 10.1016/j.jacl.2011.07.005

Doctors Data (2017). Speciality diagnostic laboratory testing. https://doctorsdata.com

Duckett, SK, Neel, JP, Fontenot, JP, & Clapham, W.M. (2009). Effects of winter stocker growth rate and finishing system on: III. Tissue proximate, fatty acid, vitamin, and cholesterol content. *J Anim Sci, 87*(9), 2961-70. doi: 10.2527/jas.2009-1850.

Dunwoody Labs (2016). *Why test diamine oxidase?* Retrieved from http://dunwoodylabs.com/index.php/profiles/intestinal-barrier-assessments-dao-hist-lps/

Environmental Working Group (2009). *Pollution in minority newborns: BPA and other cord blood pollutants.* Retrieved from http://www.ewg.org/research/minority-cord-blood-report/bpa-and-other-cord-blood-pollutants

Environmental Working Group (2015). *FDA warns of mercury in skin creams.* Retrieved from http://www.ewg.org/enviroblog/2012/03/fda-warns-mercury-skin-creams

Environmental Working Group (2017). *Get rid of the toxic dust.* Retrieved from http://www.ewg.org/research/healthy-home-tips/tip-8-get-rid-toxic-dust

Environmental Working Group (2017). *Shoppers guide to pesticides in produce.* https://www.ewg.org/foodnews/summary.php

Environmental Working Group (2017). *Shoppers guide to safe cosmetics.* http://www.ewg.org/enviroblog/2008/12/ewg-shoppers-guide-safe-cosmetics-its-easy

Fauber, J. (2014). Common diabetes medication among drugs found in Lake Michigan. *Journal Sentinel.* Retrieved from http://archive.jsonline.com/news/health/common-diabetes-medication-among-drugs-found-in-lake-michigan-b99417112z1-287238651.html

Genomix Nutrition (2017). Personalized neutrogenomic testing. https://genomixnutrition.com

Genova Diagnostics (2015). *Speciality diagnostic assessments.* https://gdx.net

Gotzsche, P.C. (2014). Our prescription drugs kill us in large numbers. *Polish Archives of Internal Medicine, 124(11),* 628-634. Retrieved from https://www.ncbi.nlm.nih.gov/pubmed/25355584

Gray, G.C. (2013). The ethics of pharmaceutical research funding: A social organization approach. *Journal of Law, Medicine & Ethics, 41*(3), 629-634.

Greenop, K.R., et al. (2013). Exposure to pesticides and the risk of childhood brain tumors. *Cancer Causes Control, 24*(7), 1269-78. doi: 10.1007/s10552-013-0205-1

Heart Math (2017). The science behind inner balanced. https://store.heartmath.com/innerbalance

Houston, M.C., Faxio, S., Chilton, F.H., Wise, D.E., Jones, K.B., Barringer, T.A., and Bramlet, D.A. (2009). *Prog Cardiovas Dis, 52*(2), 61-94. doi: 10.1016/j.pcad.2009.02.002

Houston, M. (2012). The role of nutraceutical supplements in the treatment of dyslipidemia. J Clin Hypertens, 14(2), 121-32. doi: 10.1111/j.1751-7176.2011.00576.x

Hu, F.B., and Stampfer, M.J. (1999). Nut consumption and risk of coronary heart disease: A review of epidemiological evidence. *Curr Atheroscler Rep, 1(*3), 204-9.

Huffman, K.M., et al. (2012). Exercise effects on lipids in persons with varying dietary patterns-does diet matter if they exercise? Responses in studies of a targeted risk reduction intervention through defined exercise I. Am Heart J, 164(1), 117-24. doi: 10.1016/j.ahj.2012.04.014

IGeneX (2017). Lyme disease speciality diagnostic testing. www.igenex.com

Johnson, D. (2010). Authorship and industry financial relationships: the tie that binds. *Journal of Clinical Oncology, 28*(8), 1281-1283 Retrieved from http://ascopubs.org/doi/full/10.1200/JCO.2009.26.9753

Jones, D.S.(Ed.). (2010). *Textbook of Functional Medicine.* Gig Harbor, WA: The Institute for Functional Medicine.

Kaveeshwar, S.A., and Cornwall, J. (2014). The current state of diabetes mellitus in India. Ausralasian Medical Journal, 7(1), 45-48. doi: 10.4066/AMJ.2013.1979

Kesser, C. (2010). Are you at risk for diabetes and obesity? https://chriskresser.com/are-you-at-risk-for-diabetes-and-obesity/

Kesser, C.(2017). (The diet-heart myth. http://chriskesser.com

Knutson, K.L.(2010). Sleep duration and cardio metabolic risk: a review of the epidemiological evidence. *Best Pract Res Clin Endocrinol Metab, 24*(5), 731-43. doi: 10.1016/j.beem.2010.07.001

Kris-Etherton P.M., et al. (2000). Polyunsaturated fatty acids in the food chain in the United States. *Am J Clin Nutr, 71*(1), 179S-188S. Retrieved from http:/ajcn.nutrition.org/content/71/1/179S. fullijkey=5c7af875f3dc71a303f7df78c52145e8b7c31643

Kuehn, B.M. (2010). Increased risk of ADHD associated with early exposure to pesticides, PCBs. *JAMA, 304*(1), 27-8. doi:10.1001/jama.2010.860

Lipski, E. (2012). Functional medicine/functional testing. In E. Lipski (Ed.), *Digestive Wellness*, 4th ed. (pp.109-128). New York, NY: McGraw-Hill.

Mensink, R.P., Zock, P.L., Kester, A.D., and Katan, M.B.(2003). Effects of dietary fatty acids and carbohydrates on the ratio of serum total to HDL cholesterol and on serum lipids and apolipoproteins: a meta-analysis of 60 controlled trials. Am J Clin Nutr, 77(5), 1146-55.

Merck Manual (2017). *Drug metabolism.* Retrieved from http://www.merckmanuals.com/professional/clinical-pharmacology/pharmacokinetics/drug-metabolism

Mercola, J. (2015). *What dangers are lurking in your household dust?* Retrieved from http://articles.mercola.com/sites/articles/archive/2015/09/12/household-dust-danger.aspx

Mercola, J.(2017). *Everything you need to know about intermittent fasting.* Retrieved from http://www.mercola.com/infographics/intermittent-fasting.htm

Mercola, J. (2010). Why are drug companies targeting your children as customers? Retrieved by http://articles.mercola.com/sites/articles/archive/2010/06/10/prescription-drug-use-by-us-children-on-the-rise.aspx

Mercola, J. (2013). Documentary: Pill poppers. Retrieved from http://articles.mercola.com/sites/articles/archive/2013/07/27/pill-poppers.aspx

Myers, A. (2015). The Autoimmune Solution. New York, NY: HarperCollins.

Nakazawa, D. (2008). *The Autoimmune Epidemic.* New York, NY: Simon & Schuster

National Center for Health Statistics (2017). Therapeutic drug use. Retrieved from https://www.cdc.gov/nchs/fastats/drug-use-therapeutic.htm

O'Neill, C.E., Keast, D.R., Nicklas, T.A., Fulgoni, V.L. (2011). Nut consumption is associated with decreased health risk factors for cardiovascular disease and metabolic syndrome in U.S. adults: NHANES 1999-2004. *J Am Coll Nutr, 30*(6).

Osborne, P. (2009). *What you should know about cholesterol before taking medication*. Retrieved from http://towncenterwellness.com/tag/heart-disease/

Osborne, P. (2017). Beyond Food. In P. Osborne (Ed.), *No Grain, No Pain* (pp.219-239). New York, NY: Simon & Schuster.

Park, J.D., Zheng, W.(2012). Human exposure and health effects inorganic and elemental mercury. J Prev Med Public Health, 45(6), 344-352. doi: 10.3961/jpmph.2012.45.6.344 Retrieved from https://www.ncbi.nlm.nih.gov/pmc/articles/PMC3514464/

Pesticide Action Network North America (2017). Atrazine. Retrieved from http://www.panna.org/resources/atrazine

Rakel, D. (2012). Tools for your practice. In D. Rakel (Ed.), *Integrative Medicine, 3rd ed.* (pp. 776-960). Philadelphia, PA: Elsevier Saunders.

Romm, A. (2017). http://avivaromm.com

Santos, F.L., Esteves, S.S., da Costa Pereira, A., Yancy, W.S., and Nunes, J.P. (2012). Systematic review and meta-analysis of clinical trials of the effects of low carbohydrate diet on cardiovascular risk factors. *Obes Rev, 13*(11), 1048-66. doi: 10.1111/j.1467-789X.2012.01021.x

Schneider, R.H., et al. (2012). Stress reduction in the secondary prevention of cardiovascular disease. Circulation: Cardiovascular Quality and Outcomes, 5,750-758. doi.org/10.1161/CIRCOUTCOMES.112.967406

Schramm, D.D., et al., (2003). Honey with high levels of antioxidants can provide protection to human subjects. *J Agric Food Chem, 51*(6)., 1732-5.

Seneff, S., Wainwright, G., and Mascitelli, L. (2011). Nutrition and Alzheimer's disease: The detrimental role of a high carbohydrate diet. *European Journal of Internal Medicine, 22*(2), 134-140. doi: http://dx.doi.org/10.1016/j.ejim.2010.12.017

Shaw, W. (2017). Elevated urinary glyphosate and clostridia metabolites with altered dopamine metabolism in triplets with autistic spectrum disorder or suspected seizure disorder: A case study. *Integrative Medicine,16*(1), 50-57. Retrieved from https://static1.squarespace.com/static/560ac814e4b067a33438ecea/t/58a1f7ca3a04113e81b82526/1487009743276/Shaw+IMCJ+FebMar+2017.pdf

SpectraCell Laboratories (2017). *Speciality diagnostic laboratory testing.* https://spectracell.com

Swithers, S.E. (2013). Artificial sweeteners produce the couterintuitive effect of inducing metabolic derangements. *Trends Endocrinol Metab, 24*(9), 431-41. doi: 10.1016/j.tem.2013.05.005

The Great Plains Laboratory (2017). *Enviro-Tox Panel.* https://greatplainslaboratory.com

The Huffington Post (2013). Prescription drugs: 7 out of 10 Americans take at least one, study finds. Retrieved from http://www.huffingtonpost.com/2013/06/19/prescription-drugs-prevalence-americans_n_3466801.html

The National Bureau of Economic Research (2017). Low life expectancy in the United States. Retrieved from http://www.nber.org/digest/dec09/w15213.html

Thomas, K., and Schmidt, M.S. (2012). Glaxo agrees to pay $3 billion in fraud settlement. Retrieved from http://www.nytimes.com/2012/07/03/business/glaxosmithkline-agrees-to-pay-3-billion-in-fraud-settlement.html

United Mitochondrial Disease Foundation (2017): *Understanding mitochondrial disease.* Retrieved from https://www.umdf.org/what-is-mitochondrial-disease/

United States Department of Health and Human Services, Office of Disease Prevention and Health Promotion (2014). National action plan for adverse drug event prevention. Washington, DC. Retrieved from https://health.gov/hcq/pdfs/ade-action-plan-508c.pdf

United States Environmental Protection Agency (EPA) (2016). *How people are exposed to mercury.* Retrieved from https://www.epa.gov/mercury/how-people-are-exposed-mercury

Vigues, S., Dotson, C.D., and Munger, S.D. (2009). The receptor basis of sweet taste in animals. Results Probl Cell Differ, 47, 187-202. doi: 10.1007/400_2008_2

Vreugdenhill, A.C.E., et al., (2001). LPS-binding protein circulated in association with apoB-containing lipoproteins and enhances endotoxin-LDL/VLDL interaction. *J Clin Invest, 107*(2), 225-234. doi: 10.1172/JCI10832

Wagstaff, A. (2014). Big Pharma has higher profit margins than any other industry. Retrieved from https://www.andruswagstaff.com/blog/big-pharma-has-higher-profit-margins-than-any-other-industry

Wentz, I. (2017). Protocols for removing toxins. In I. Wentz (Ed.), *Hashimoto's Protocol.* (pp.331-353). New York, NY: HarperCollins.

White, J.S. (2008). Straight talk about high-fructose corn syrup: what it is and what it ain't. Am J Clin Nutr, 88(6), 1716S-1721S. doi: 10.3945/ajcn.2008.25825B

World Mercury Project (2017): Hiding in plain site: Mercury still lurks in many common pharmaceutical products. Retrieved from https://worldmercuryproject.org/hiding-plain-sight-mercury-still-lurks-many-common-pharmaceutical-products/

Worthington, V. (2001). Nutritional quality of organic versus conventional fruits, vegetables, and grains. *Journal of Alternative and Complementary Medicine, 7*(2), 161-173. Retrieved from http://ucanr.edu/datastoreFiles/608-794.pdf

Yamagishi, K., et al., (2009). Dietary intake of saturated fatty acids and mortality from cardiovascular disease in Japanese: the Japan Collaborative Cohort Study of Evaluation of Cancer Risk. *Am J Clin Nutri, 92*(4). doi: 10.3945/ajcn.2009.29146

Yusuf, S., et al., (2004). Effect of potentially modifiable risk factors associated with myocardial infarction in 52 countries (the INTERHEART study): case-control study. *Lancet, 364*(9438), 937-52.

Zhong, W., et al. (2013). Age and ses patterns of drug prescribing in a defined American population. *Mayo Clin Proc, 88*(7), 697-707. Retrieved from http://www.mayoclinicproceedings.org/article/S0025-6196(13)00357-1/pdf

ZRT Labs (2017). *Specialty hormone lab testing.* http://zrtlab.com

ABOUT THE AUTHOR

CHERYL WINTER, MS APRN, FNP-BC, BC-ADM, IFMCP, MS RDN, CDE

Cheryl holds two Master of Science (M.S.) degrees, one in Nutrition and Food Sciences that led to her becoming a Registered Dietitian/Nutritionist. The other M.S. degree in Nursing led to Cheryl's Advanced Practice Registered Nurse status and subsequently her Board Certification as a Family Nurse Practitioner. She also has Board Certification in Advanced Diabetes Management and is a Certified Diabetes Educator.

Cheryl is also a certified practitioner with the prestigious Institute for Functional Medicine and is currently pursuing a Doctorate of Clinical Nutrition from Maryland University of Integrative Health. She is also co-author of the book, *Diet Therapy in Advanced Practice Nursing,* published by McGraw-Hill.

As the creator of the "GET Balanced, Fit & Slim Step-Power® Transformation" Program, Cheryl helps clients worldwide (virtually and in-office) with her healing methods that allows them to kick disease in the butt & live life to the fullest.

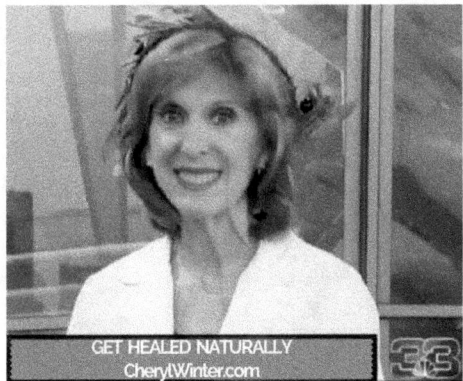

GET HEALED NATURALLY
CherylWinter.com

Cheryl can help you, too, reverse, prevent, and/or eliminate all types of chronic disease without drugs. You can discover more about her and her work at the following websites:

http://CherylWinter.com

http://DiabeteStepsRx.com

http://GetHealedNaturally.com

www.ingramcontent.com/pod-product-compliance
Lightning Source LLC
Chambersburg PA
CBHW072138270326
41931CB00010B/1794